EMOTIONAL UNDERSTANDING

Emotional Understanding

STUDIES IN PSYCHOANALYTIC EPISTEMOLOGY

Donna M. Orange

THE GUILFORD PRESS
New York   London

© 1995 The Guilford Press
A Division of Guilford Publications, Inc.
72 Spring Street, New York, NY 10012

Printed in the United States of America

This book is printed on acid-free paper.

Last digit is print number: 9 8 7 6 5 4 3 2 1

Library of Congress Cataloging-in-Publication Data

Orange, Donna M.
    Emotional understanding : studies in psychoanalytic
    epistemology / Donna M. Orange.
        p. cm.
    Includes bibliographical references and index.
    ISBN 1-57230-010-8
    1. Psychoanalysis and philosophy. 2. Comprehension
(Theory of knowledge) 3. Comprehension. I. Title.
BF175.4.P45O73   1995
150.19′5—dc20   95-34661
                                                    CIP

Excerpt from "The Longing" is used by permission of Doubleday, a division of
Bantam Doubleday Dell Publishing Group, Inc. ©1962 by Beatrice Roethke,
Administratrix of the Estate of Theodore Roethke, from *The Collected Poems of
Theodore Roethke* by Theodore Roethke.

Earlier versions of some chapters appeared in the following publications: Chap-
ter 4, in *New Therapeutic Visions: Progress in Self Psychology* (Vol. 8), and Chapter
12, in *Freud's Case Studies: Self Psychological Perspectives*, both published by The
Analytic Press; Chapter 5, in *The Widening Scope of Self Psychology*, published by
The Analytic Press, and in *The Intersubjective Perspective*, published by Jason
Aronson. All are adapted by permission.

For all psychoanalytic fallibilists,
especially Bernie

Acknowledgments

Many people have helped me write this book, whether or not they will agree with what I have said. Each of them has transformed "constructive criticism" from an oxymoron into a process of understanding, of making sense together.

For helpful readings of parts or all of the manuscript in different phases of its development, I thank Margaret Andrews, Mary Anker, George Atwood, Howard Bacal, Andrine Baker, Kathleen Fischer, James Fosshage, Natalie Gannon, Jill Gentile, Judith Glassgold, Jacqueline Gotthold, Patricia Horn, Peter Lessem, Frances Madden, Anna Ornstein, Henry Pinsker, Robert Stolorow, and Peter Thomson. Each has been a thoughtful reader and a great support in ways too individual to explain. Some—Jackie Gotthold, Peter Lessem, and especially George Atwood—have read several versions and have generally suffered through this process with me. Kitty Moore, my editor at Guilford, suggested that I write a book, nursed the project along, and rescued me from some of my tendency toward pedantry. Claudia Kohner has gone far beyond the normal copy editor's duties in helping me to make this book readable. I give what the Dutch call "heartfelt thanks" to all of you. Nevertheless, the opinions, omissions, and outright mistakes in this book remain mine.

I also need to thank and acknowledge all those whose thoughts or expressions I have unwittingly borrowed without citation. I will borrow again, this time consciously, from the words of Winnicott (1965):

I wish to acknowledge my debt to my psycho-analytic colleagues. I have grown up as a member of the group, and after so many years of interrelating it is now impossible for me to know what I have learned and what I have contributed. The writings of any one of us must be to some extent plagiaristic. Nevertheless I think we do not copy: we work and observe and think and discover, even if it can be shown that what we discover has been discovered before. (p. 11)

In this statement, Winnicott rejected the concern with priority and articulated the notion of the community of scholars. My group within the community of scholars is the Institute for the Psycho-analytic Study of Subjectivity, which explicitly intends to be such a collaborative community, devoted to the development of psycho-analytic theory and practice. I thank everyone connected with the institute for being part of the community in which I could "grow up" and start to feel able to contribute. I am also grateful to those patients who gave me permission to write about them and about our process of making sense together. Finally I thank my supervisees, my students, and especially all my patients for teaching me understanding.

Contents

CHAPTER 1

Introduction: Making Sense Together

> The person with understanding does not
> know and judge as one who stands apart and
> unaffected; but rather, as one united by a
> specific bond with the other, he thinks with
> the other and undergoes the situation with
> him.
> —HANS-GEORG GADAMER, *Truth and Method*

*T*his book is a series of studies in psychoanalytic epistemology. Epistemology, the inquiry into the nature and limits of human knowledge, has been undergoing a transformation toward increased humility because we recognize that our knowledge of anything is perspectival and thus necessarily incomplete. Similarly, this work of psychoanalytic epistemology replaces the questions "What can we know?" and "How can we be certain that we know?" with the queries "What is psychoanalytic understanding?" and "How does such understanding heal emotional wounds?" This shift reflects many recent changes in psychoanalytic thinking: from drive to the organization of experience as primary motivator, from scientific objectivism to hermeneutic perspectivism, from seeing psychoanalysis as hard science to finding it among the humanities or human sciences, and, above all, from the values of independence and isolation to those of interdependence and community.

The central thesis of this book is that psychoanalytic understanding emerges from mutual participation—primarily emotional participation—in the intersubjective field formed by the two subjectivities of patient and therapist. The process of struggling for and reaching good-enough understanding can heal emotional wounds and alter a person's organized experiencing.

PSYCHOANALYSIS AND PHILOSOPHY

Studies in psychoanalytic epistemology are necessarily interdisciplinary. I bring to this undertaking my years of studying and teaching philosophy, and those spent studying psychology and in psychoanalytic training and practice. This book, therefore, is a kind of discussion between the philosophical and clinical parts of me, an open conversation that the reader is invited to join. We will examine some aspect of psychoanalytic understanding in each chapter, entertaining hypotheses about the nature, function, and limits of such understanding. Many questions will remain open, standing as invitations to further study.

This book consists of studies, from various perspectives, of aspects of psychoanalytic understanding. It forms a sort of tapestry in which the threads reveal a picture of psychoanalysis as patient and analyst making sense together, reaching an emotional understanding. I begin with the most general nature of understanding and examine the conditions for the possibility of understanding, psychoanalytic or otherwise. In the middle chapters I advocate what I call "perspectival realism," a revised view of countertransference, and a conception of experience as both given and made. These ideas are crucial components of any adequate psychoanalytic epistemology. In the later chapters I adopt a more clinical perspective on understanding, and I suggest that the only sort of understanding that can heal emotional wounds and integrate human experiencing is emotional understanding. Throughout I rely on both philosophical and clinical thinking to explain the ideas under discussion.

Historically, however, the relationship between psychoanalysis and philosophy has not been one of mutual respect. Freud stated that "the delusions of paranoiacs have an unpalatable external similarity and internal kinship to the systems of our philosophers" (1919, p. 161), and he claimed that "We have nothing to expect from philosophy except that it will once again haughtily point out to us the intellectual inferiority of the object of our study" (1915–1916, pp. 97–98). The philosopher Grunbaum (1984) denounces psychoanalytic pretensions to scientific status and suggests that psychoanalysis generally is intellectually incoherent. Part of the unfriendliness between philosophy and psychoanalysis may come from occupational distance. Philosophy lives in the university and psychoanalysis in free-standing institutes and consulting rooms. Nevertheless, both disciplines belong to the humanities (Kohut, 1985), and both have formed me. So readers of this book will find an interdisciplinary inquiry or "conversation" that writers in either field might not undertake. Plato defined thinking as a conversation "that the mind carries on with itself about any subject it is considering" (*Theatetus*, 189e), and I describe analysis as conversation, as making sense together. In addition, I believe that a dialogue between philosophy and psychoanalysis can reach some useful descriptions of the nature of psychoanalytic understanding.

In this conversation I argue for holding some basic attitudes. The first attitude places a value on theory-choice and theory-improvement. This concern reflects the philosopher's commitment to the examined life, to acknowledging the fundamental conceptual presuppositions or assumptions embedded in our clinical theories and in our work. A second value or attitude concerns the importance of fallibilism, the commitment to hold theory lightly, to live with uncertainty and ambiguity, and to be always prepared to revise our views. This attitude keeps us constantly ready to learn something, from our patients and from each other.

In addition to these methodological attitudes, I argue for an epistemology that I call "perspectival realism." "Objectivism"—the assumption that the known is independent of the knower—and "relativism"—Hegel's night in which all cows are black (nothing is distinguishable)—are equally poor alternatives. Nevertheless, psychoanalysis—in theory and in practice—can move "beyond objectivism and relativism" (Bernstein, 1983) in the direction of a perspectival or dialogical realism. Such a moderate realism acknowledges the constructivist critique with its insistence on the contribution of the subject or subjects to the making of meaning, but it rejects the turn toward relativism. In accord with fallibilism, it recognizes that each person's perspective is inevitably partial and that a more adequate view of anything requires dialogue. In such conversation we attempt to reach, practically speaking, a good-enough understanding of whatever is under discussion. In psychoanalysis, where the subject matter is a person's emotional life, understanding that heals requires a mutually experienced emotional connection between patient and analyst.

This view of psychoanalytic understanding raises additional questions. We must ask what conditions and attitudes support good-enough emotional understanding. One requirement is the emotional availability of a particular analyst for a healing connection with the particular person who comes for therapy or analysis. This implies the willingness and ability of the therapist to provide for that person a developmental second chance at a rich and integrated emotional life. A second condition is that analyst and patient embrace an enriched conception of memory that includes tacit and somatic forms as well as verbal expressions. To acknowledge such knowing-beyond-words requires a radical questioning of empiricist assumptions and of commonly accepted theories of truth and knowledge.

EPISTEMOLOGY AND INTERSUBJECTIVITY

An adequate psychoanalytic epistemology must eschew individualism and the myth of the isolated mind (Stolorow & Atwood, 1992), and it must move toward both subjective and intersubjective conceptions of understanding. In ordinary discourse we distinguish subjective understanding from knowing-about. Knowing-about is external and observational. Understanding is knowledge by participation, in the Platonic sense, knowledge from within. For example, there is an enormous difference between knowing-about the Hopi Indian culture and understanding life as a Hopi would, or between knowing-about the French language and understanding French. An ill friend recently told me, "You know, but you don't understand, because you have always been healthy." For Kohut (1959), the only kind of knowing that could count as psychoanalytic was knowledge from within, understanding gained by introspection and empathy (or vicarious introspection). While we can know something about human beings through social psychology or neuropsychology, according to Kohut, understanding can only be achieved through empathy.

Intersubjectivity theory (Stolorow, Brandchaft, & Atwood, 1987) refines this view by clarifying the notion of "within." Psychoanalytic understanding is knowledge gained from inside the intersubjective field formed by the intersection of two differently organized subjectivities. In dialogue, both participants attempt to expand their original subjective perspectives to take in, comprehend, and understand more of the other's experience. We do this, as Kohut and other self psychologists have shown, by placing ourselves, as consistently as we can, in the other's shoes, both cognitively and emotionally. We understand by attempting to participate in the emotional experience, in the being, of the other.

In this book's exploration of psychoanalytic epistemology, "understanding" will primarily mean an intersubjective process of emotional comprehension, of reaching or developing an understanding with another. When a bright and appealing young scholar consults me during a bout of profound depression after a series of puzzling academic failures, we struggle together to find the source of the trouble. I call this process understanding. The older psychoanalytic notion of interpretation fails to capture the intersubjective nature of this ordinary clinical process, and it underestimates the influence of the observer's capacities and assumptions on the extent and kind of understanding reached. An analyst must be Gadamer's "person with understanding," able and willing to enter the patient's suffering and share the painful history, able and willing to "undergo the situation" with the other. I will call this combination of capacity and willingness "emotional availability." Only when it is present can patient and analyst make sense of what seems senseless—my bright and usually successful young scholar's deep depression and suicidal feelings, for example.

The term "understanding" thus refers to both person and process, to both self and relation. The individual comprehends, or takes in, the relation, while the relationship includes, and partly forms, the experiencing and experienced self. Forcing a choice between self and relatedness maintains a false dualism that undermines both psychoanalytic treatment and theory. In emotional development, the requirement to choose between ties to caretakers and development of an articulated self can be pathogenic (Brandchaft, 1994). Similarly, the choice in theory between "I" and "we" may result in forms of blindness. Intersubjectivity theory gives equal weight to the "I" and to the "we," treats them as inextricably linked, and thereby offers the best opportunity thus far to comprehend psychoanalytic understanding.

MAKING SENSE TOGETHER

Conceptualizing psychoanalysis as "making sense together," both raises and presumes partial answers to fundamental questions addressed in this book. What goes into making sense? Fact? Theory? And what are these? Of what do we make sense? Reality? Fantasy? Or what? I will argue that psychoanalysis is primarily a collaborative effort to comprehend a person's emotional experience. Such comprehension means entering into and dwelling inside the experience of the patient, including the experience of the analytic relationship, by both partners. Together patient and analyst struggle to make sense of the patient's experience of being the person she or he is, particularly but not exclusively in the analytic relationship.

Making sense is an affair of memory, emotion, and anticipation, of past, present, and future. Paradoxically, it sometimes includes the recognition that some events make no sense in any perspective available to humans. Making sense stretches the bounds of traditional bivalued logic and forces us to think about experience in more holistic, but less neat, categories. It teaches respect for the "unthought known" (Bollas, 1987), but it makes us endlessly curious about it. Psychoanalysis can generate such curiosity if it can foster comfort with uncertainty and unfinished business. In Rilke's (1934) words, one ought to "be patient toward all that is unsolved in your heart, and to try to love the questions themselves like locked rooms and like books that are written in a very foreign tongue" (p. 35). "Making sense" is a way of connecting to the uncharted and mysterious parts of ourselves and of one another.

The urge to make sense is distinctively human. We find some capacity to organize in all living beings, perhaps even in inanimate nature. Higher forms of life show increasing capacity for feeling, and more flexibility and complexity in their ways of organizing experience. Healthy humans have a developing and lifelong propensity to reflect, to organize experience variously, and especially to wonder or converse about meanings.

Psychoanalysis is a special conversation about meaning; it is an attempt of analyst and patient to make sense together of the patient's emotional life. In Gadamer's (1991) phrase, we undergo the situation together (p. 288), especially in the transference and countertransference (or cotransference, see Chapter 5). In Hoffman's (1993) words, "I see our intimate involvement with, and commitment to, our patients as requiring that we be partners with them in their struggles with often agonizing existential choices and predicaments" (p. 19). We make sense of a person's life by feeling it together and reflecting on it together in the intersubjective field of treatment.

INTERSUBJECTIVITY, SELF PSYCHOLOGY, AND PSYCHOANALYTIC UNDERSTANDING

My philosophical perspective on psychoanalytic issues has caused me to lean toward the intersubjective view of psychoanalysis because it views understanding as the means to and the goal of successful psychoanalysis. Intersubjectivity, in this book, refers broadly to the psychoanalytic theory articulated in the work of Atwood and Stolorow (1984), and developed both in Stolorow, Brandchaft, and Atwood (1987) and in Stolorow and Atwood (1992). For these authors, any two or more subjectivities may make up an intersubjective field. In childhood or in analysis the interplay of child and parent or of patient and analyst produces its own psychological configurations, and these form a system. Psychoanalysis goes beyond individual subjectivity and seeks to understand the workings of this system and its effect on an individual's way of organizing experience.

Intersubjectivity theory describes the emergence and modification of subjectivity, and it defines these processes as irreducibly relational. This book is a development of intersubjectivity theory, modifying that theory to emphasize the emotional dimension of human understanding. My idiom—a woman's voice, perhaps—provides a more explicit emphasis on emotional life, emotional connection, emotional memory, and emotional understanding.

I want to distinguish my use of the terms "intersubjective" and "intersubjectivity" from two related ideas. First, by "intersubjective" I mean a relatedness that can contain any two people to the extent that they have become subjects, without regard to developmental level. My use of the term differs from that of Daniel Stern (1985), who, in his description of infant development, defines intersubjectivity as the attainment of the ability to recognize another's subjectivity as connected to one's own. In contrast, this recognition by a patient may be a comparatively late achievement in the intersubjective field of an analysis, especially for patients such as those described by Guntrip (1969) and Kohut (1971), yet the intersubjective field exists from the onset of the analysis.

Second, although both intersubjectivity theory and interpersonalism are relational theories, they differ. Interpersonal theory often concerns itself with who is doing what to whom, focusing on concepts such as gambits, control, agency, and responsibility. Because the analyst maintains an external perspective, doing interpersonalist work can interfere with the ability to undergo the situation *with* the patient (Gadamer, 1991). Although intersubjectivity theory may at times focus on the *experience* of control and agency, it resembles more closely those currents in relational thinking that emphasize development within a caregiving situation (Winnicott, 1958; Bollas, 1987; Ghent, 1992) and the exchange of differently organized and positioned perspectives (Aron, 1992).

On one side, an intersubjective point of view transcends the Freudian view of human beings as self-contained bundles of better or more poorly harnessed sexual and aggressive instincts that are directed at "objects." Intersubjectivity theory sees humans as organizers of experience, as subjects. Therefore, it views psychoanalytic treatment as the dialogic attempt of two people to understand one person's organization of emotional experience by "making sense together" of their shared experience.

On the other hand, my version of intersubjectivity theory lives comfortably with self psychology, another relational theory and my original psychoanalytic home. By speaking of selfobject experience or selfobject relatedness, self psychology explains how a patient can use the special intersubjective field of treatment to form or heal self-experience. In treatment, we offer patients a developmental "second chance" at a secure emotional attachment. Within such a bond they can experience the primary selfobject relatedness needed to develop a strong and valued sense of self.

The psychoanalytic understanding I examine here provides and works through this emotional "new beginning" (A. Ornstein, 1991) for the patient. Interpretive work, seen as a collaborative project of making sense together of a patient's emotional life, both supports and creates the healing selfobject experience. Understanding, in this view, is a relational form of healing. Self psychology describes the intersubjective field of treatment as a form of relatedness in which an analyst or therapist can be unequivocally on the patient's side (Tolpin, 1991), entering and remaining with the patient's self and relational experience. We do this, of course, through our cotransference (Orange, 1994)—including our personal history and the "sense of things" we have inferred from it—and from our training and theories.

In addition, the attention self psychology gives to the effects of relational deprivation and of trauma concretely shapes my clinical thinking. No other psychoanalytic theory, I believe, focuses so directly on the emotional suffering and confusion of patients. No matter what level of abstraction or generality my theorizing may reach, self psychology keeps me emotionally close to patients.

However, intersubjectivity theory, as I conceive it, functions at a different level of discourse from that of self psychology. It describes the triadic system or field in *any* psychoanalytic treatment, classical or relational. The emotional organizing principles that each participant has distilled from relational experience form the two subjectivities. The interplay of these two subjectivities forms the third element of the intersubjective triad. While intersubjectivity theory has clinical implications that require the analyst to be sensitive to the triad, this does not mean that the relationship is a reified entity separate from the two subjectivities. Instead the concept of a "triad" highlights the capacity of the field itself to have both history and emotional qualities.[*]

I find intersubjectivity a productive metatheory. As a cognitive

---

[*]Ogden (1994) has presented a similar idea.

framework, it helps me to comprehend some differences among the metapsychologies and clinical approaches of various psychoanalytic theories. (Chapter 3, "Theory-Choice and Fallibilism," will show how this works.) My organizing principles, however, which lead me to see developing emotional life as a central value, make me, in practice, a self psychologist. I hope this book contributes to the growth and development of both self psychology and intersubjectivity theory, neither of which I can do without.

I also hope that this book becomes a participant in the larger psychoanalytic conversation. A major contribution by Greenberg and Mitchell (1983), developed by Mitchell (1988, 1993), has both identified and participated in a widespread shift toward relational theories of human nature, psychopathology, and cure. This change has revolutioned the conception of psychoanalytic understanding, and its influence continues to develop in several schools of thought.

Interpersonalists (e.g., Hoffman 1983, 1991, 1992a, 1992b; Donnel Stern, 1992) are developing relational theories under the aegis of social constructivism. This view offers a relativist or contextualist epistemology as an alternative to the empiricism and positivism inherent in classical psychoanalysis and ego psychology. Meanwhile, the British independent school—which originally included Fairbairn, Guntrip, Winnicott, Balint, and Bowlby—continues to grow in the work of Bollas (1987, 1989). Bollas's contributions on memory and personal idiom place him, along with the self psychologists, among those thinkers Ghent (1992) calls the developmental–relational theorists. Self psychology, given context by the intersubjectivity theory of Stolorow et al. (1987), has adopted a phenomenological view of the nature of psychoanalytic understanding (Kohut, 1959; P. Ornstein & A. Ornstein, 1985). I am indebted to all of these thinkers—and to those (Brandchaft, 1986; Bacal & Newman, 1990) who have identified the relationships among some of these theories—in my attempt to understand psychoanalytic understanding.

To repeat, my studies in psychoanalytic epistemology aim to present a view of psychoanalysis as emotional understanding that is philosophically defensible and clinically creative. First, I will argue that my psychoanalytic epistemology involves replacing both objectivism and relativism with a perspectival realism. Second, I believe that in our theoretical and clinical studies we need to replace dogmatism and the search for certainty with a thorough-going fallibilism, the attitude of holding our own opinions lightly. In psychoanalysis this attitude has probably been best exemplified historically by Sandor Ferenczi, who was always ready to say he had been wrong, and currently by Bernard Brandchaft. Third, I believe we need to balance and integrate any cognitive cast in psychoanalysis with a clear commitment to the attempt at healing the emotional life of human beings. Finally, I believe psychoanalysis needs to continue its recent efforts to replace all forms of "one-body" or "isolated mind" (Stolorow & Atwood, 1992) psychology with fully relational and intersubjective accounts of human nature and motivation. In this spirit I describe psychoanalysis as emotional understanding gained by "making sense together." Only together with our patients, and with each other, can we make sense in our clinical work and in our search for better theory.

Psychoanalysis is therapy by understanding. It seeks to promote comprehension and to heal by participation in the emotional life of human beings. Psychoanalytic understanding is making sense *together*.

CHAPTER 2

Understanding Understanding[*]

My real love is new understanding.
—HEINZ KOHUT

Sometimes to understand the present, one
needs to study the past.
—Chinese fortune cookie, quoted in
RICHARD BERNSTEIN, *The New Constellation*

*M*ost people enter analysis, or psychoanalytic forms of therapy, baffled by themselves. Their feelings, reactions, behavior, inhibitions, and difficulties in relating make no sense to them. Even worse, early caretakers have often convinced these patients that they are beyond understanding. Our efforts to "make sense together," to engage these patients in a process of understanding themselves and their relationships, often amazes them. "You always think there are reasons for what I do or feel," a young woman said to me with considerable surprise.

If psychoanalytic understanding is as central to the healing process as I believe it is, it deserves our serious inquiry into its nature. On the assumption that ideas develop historically, this

---

[*]I had entitled this chapter long before I saw *On Understanding Understanding* (1994) by the late Vincent G. Potter. Potter directed my 1979 dissertation on Charles Sanders Peirce, and he must have influenced my thinking more than I had realized.

chapter provides an intellectual genealogy for the idea of understanding, and it maps the path through Kohut's conceptualization
of empathy into psychoanalytic understanding as a way of knowing
together and being together.

Psychoanalysis was born at a particular moment in intellectual
and cultural history. This moment contained a tension between
faith in causality and the search for meaning. Freud's work included both a "Project for a Scientific Psychology" (1895), which
was an attempt to establish physiological causes for all mental
phenomena, and a lifelong effort to explore the meanings of
puzzling human experience. This tension persists to this day in
psychoanalysis as a division between those who regard psychoanalysis as a science—usually organized around the conception of
instinctual drives—and those who see it as an interpretive, or
hermeneutic, and relational enterprise. Mitchell's (Greenberg &
Mitchell, 1983; Mitchell, 1988, 1993) work delineates a broad and
deep shift toward the latter point of view.

I believe that the intersubjective conception (Stolorow et al.,
1987) of psychoanalytic understanding not only makes a place for
but also does justice to both points of view. The intersubjective
approach shares the generality of scientific inquiry and the particularity of empathic concentration on one individual's organized
and organizing subjective world. Although, like other relational
theories, an intersubjective perspective gives clear primacy to
subjective meaning over objective "reality," it appreciates both the
particularity of organized emotional experience and the generality
of humanness, thus providing a balanced context for our epistemological inquiry into the nature of understanding.

THE HISTORY OF UNDERSTANDING

The modern notion of understanding came into philosophy with
Kant's (1781) *Critique of Pure Reason,* which questioned the grounds
for claiming to know any external reality. To save knowledge—especially scientific knowledge—from his own critique, Kant distinguished pure reason (*Vernunft*) from understanding (*Verstand*).
Understanding, based on what Kant called "the categories" (structures or organizers of experience), yields no absolutes, no things-

in-themselves beyond the reach of human experience, and no extraexperiential deity. Although Kant found it reasonable to *believe* in real moral differences and in a deity—the pragmatists were his legitimate heirs—he confined *understanding* to experiential phenomena. Understanding seeks to unify and organize more direct experience, and it gives us categories for doing so. In Kant's view, what we already understand determines what we can come to understand. We owe to him our contemporary awareness of the ways our theories and preconceptions shape and limit our perception.

Hegel criticized the Kantian notion of understanding as being too limited by its fixed categories and its devotion to abstraction. Only by dialectical thinking, Hegel thought, could we overcome the inadequacies of the categories of understanding and thereby proceed by reason or speculative philosophy to know the whole. He believed that finite understanding derives meaning only from the infinite, or absolute totality. Reacting against such views, Nietzsche rejected both finite understanding and Hegel's totality in favor of antirationality, paradox, and eternal recurrence.

It was left to Dilthey (1989) and the hermeneutic philosophers to rehabilitate understanding. Eschewing metaphysics and comprehensive world views, they attempted the more modest task of examining the process of understanding. Dilthey distinguished the *Naturwissenschaften* (natural sciences) from the *Geisteswissenschaften* (cultural sciences), among which he included law, economics, literature, art, philosophy, and psychology. These disciplines require understanding from within, understanding through flexible categories drawn from the personal lived experience (*Erlebnis*) of interaction in a social milieu. Understanding means the use of such categories to penetrate beyond the obvious into the life of a person, the inner spirit of historical epochs, and the meanings and purposes expressed by law, economics, or historical events. Since such understanding depends on self-knowledge in historical context, it can never be complete. Instead, this kind of knowing is a constant approximation of what we seek to know.

For Dilthey, understanding is not a purely cognitive enterprise. We can explain nature, identify causes of observed effects, but we seek to *understand* human beings. Understanding consists of reexperiencing or sharing the experience of the world as another experiences it. Dilthey's view of understanding resembles Kohut's (1959) definition of empathy as vicarious introspection.

Heidegger moved beyond Dilthey by situating the knower squarely in the known. Heidegger's *Dasein*, or being-in-the-world, offered a compelling alternative to the detached objectivism and positivism of modern science, and it included the observer within what is to be observed. Like Kant's categories, Heidegger's "fore-conceptions" spotlighted the observer's contribution to all understanding.

It was only another short step to Gadamer's (1991) "dialogic" conception of understanding. According to this view, interpretation no longer defines the field of hermeneutics; instead the deeper, broader, and more fundamental process of understanding does. Interpretation can be, as Winnicott (1965, p. 189) explained, a means to test the limits of our understanding and to find our way together beyond these limits. Nevertheless, one person gives another an interpretation. Understanding, on the contrary, emerges from the work/play of two or more people together. Understanding is a *relational* way of being and knowing.

Gadamer's view of understanding has several important features. Play may be the most important element of his view of understanding. While Gadamer often speaks of the effort of understanding and of hermeneutic work, he clearly asks that we approach it in a playful spirit, with an openness to letting the other say something new to us. A kind of dialogical volleyball, between tradition and future, between self and other, between question and supposition, creates a field in which something new can emerge from the interplay of subjectivities. (Thus Gadamer escapes from the Kantian prison in which we can understand only what we already understand.) In psychoanalysis I think such play is not restricted to dream analysis but, if the emotional atmosphere is safe enough, can even be part of the analysis of ruptures and misunderstandings. "I wonder what is going on with us? We aren't usually like this."

Simultaneously, Gadamer believes (1979) that all understanding is ultimately self-understanding. We can understand another only through the perspective of our personal organized subjectivity. For hermeneutic understanding there is no blank screen, no neutrality, no anonymity. In Gadamer's view, we understand by standing under or within, not outside. In other words, to understand we try to enter not the isolated mind (Stolorow & Atwood, 1992) of the other but the whole emotional predicament in which the other has formed a point of view or has organized experience. This must be something like what Kohut meant when he spoke of understanding in depth, which referred not so much to a topographical search, or mental spelunking, but to the understanding of "complex mental states" (1978c, pp. 579–580). The self-understanding required for any comprehension involves this entry, through our own perspective, into the perspective of the other. Understanding, according to Gadamer, "is not an act of subjectivity, but proceeds from the commonality that binds us to a tradition" (p. 293). Like Sullivan (1953), who reminded us that "we are all more simply human than otherwise" (p. 32), Gadamer denies that we can understand from a distance. Similarly, when a patient asks, "Does any of this make sense to you?" I can say yes only if I can feel some kinship with the patient's struggles.

Nevertheless, the other is other. The interplay, for Gadamer, between the commonality/familiarity and the strangeness of the historically situated other is the space of understanding. "The true locus of hermeneutics is this in-between" (1991, p. 295). As a result, no method, technique, or procedure will yield understanding. We must have the courage to stand under or within the other, to play with the other, to allow understanding to emerge between us.

Ricoeur (1979), too, recognizes the "nonmethodic," or emergent, character of understanding:

> Strictly speaking, only explanation is methodic. Understanding is rather the nonmethodic moment which, in the sciences of interpretation, comes together with the methodic moment of explanation. Understanding precedes, accompanies, closes, and thus envelops explanation. In return explanation develops understanding analytically. (p. 165)

Perhaps it is because explanation can be methodic that analysts have given so much attention to the correctness of interpretations and to their proper sequencing, surface to depth, for example. Method provides a sense of security and a safe emotional distance, both from the patient and from our own emotional responses. The price we may pay for these protections is the sacrifice of understanding for explanation. In contrast, empathy, a necessary but not sufficient condition for understanding, is nonmethodical and fallible. Unlike Gadamer, who replaces empathy with understanding, I believe that empathic participation in the emotional life of the other makes the interplay of psychoanalytic understanding possible. To study psychoanalytic epistemology, therefore, we must examine the nature and function of empathy.

EMPATHY AND UNDERSTANDING

Although the term "empathy" is common currency in conversation among mental health professionals, its meaning is woefully unclear. Comparatively new as an English word, it is a translation of the German *Einfuhlung,* which literally means "a feeling into." Many thinkers have attempted to define empathy. Weigert (1962), for example, cites Max Scheler's "empathy as a form of emotional contagion based on a process of identification." Hobson (1985) notes that "empathy" was first used in esthetics to denote the appreciation of a work of art. The word's meaning then broadened to include expressed "appreciation of what another person is experiencing at this moment" (p. 10). Hobson comments further that we often think of empathy as a one-way process, but that instead it means a step toward mutuality or conversation. This suggestion is close to the view of Harry Stack Sullivan, as reported by Fromm-Reichmann (1950), that "empathy" refers to a nonverbal "communion between people" (p. 30). Sullivan—and later Winnicott (1965)—believed that empathy originated in the preverbal infant–caretaker relationship.

Here, however, let us look at the assumptions underlying these definitions and examine empathy as a kind of knowledge. Eager to free empathy from associations with sentimentality and sympathy, Kohut (1959; 1971) claimed that empathy was the primary—perhaps the only—epistemological method proper to psychoanalysis. Therapists, he thought, know by empathy—"a major instrument of psychoanalytic observation" (1971, p. 37)—the experience and history of others. Empathy, for Kohut (1977), is "vicarious introspection," the capacity to place oneself, both cognitively and emotionally, in another's shoes, to see or hear from another's perspective. Empathy, Kohut (1971) held, "is a mode of cognition which is specifically attuned to the perception of complex psychological configurations" (p. 300). Kohut emphasized that empathy is not equivalent to sympathy, viewing empathy, instead, as a tool for data collection. Yet, he cautioned against relying solely on empathy:

> The scientific psychologist, in general, and the psychoanalyst in particular, not only must have free access to empathic understanding; they must also be able to relinquish the empathic attitude. If they cannot be empathic, they cannot observe and collect the data which they need: if they cannot step beyond empathy, they cannot set up hypotheses and theories, and thus, ultimately cannot achieve explanations. (1971, p. 303)

In his last paper, however, Kohut (1981) qualified the distinction between empathy and explanation. He came to view explanation as a higher form of empathy, analogous to the mother's shift from physical contact to facially expressed pride in her child's achievement: "from a lower form of empathy to a higher form of empathy" (p. 532). Although Kohut's "empathy" stopped short of the mutuality found in an intersubjective conception of understanding, it did involve a relational mode of knowing emotional reality.

What is this mode of cognition that Kohut called empathy? To offer an answer that retains Kohut's idea and still does justice to the other understandings of empathy described above, we must reach back into the history of philosophy. Scientific empiricism, with its sharp distinction between objective scientifically verifiable fact and subjective experience, will give us no help. This tradition sets up certainty as a criterion of knowledge. It prescribes tests of verifiability like those common in the "hard" sciences (Carnap, 1936; Hempel, 1951). This view excludes from the realm of knowledge such unquantifiable matters as a person's own history and the experience of another's subjectivity (the notorious problem of other minds). Kohut (1984) criticized this conception of scientific objectivity, pointing out that even small-particle physics both posits an irreducible interaction of observer and observed and illustrates the uncertainty principle (cf.

Sucharov, 1994). *A fortiori* in psychoanalysis, we must consider the influence of the observing subject.

Until Hume's (1739) *A Treatise of Human Nature,* philosophers regarded some matters not accessible to empirical testing as knowable. For these pre-Humean thinkers, such "unscientific" matters were more knowable though less fully known than the more easily verifiable facts (Aquinas, 1265–1273). Examination of these earlier epistemological–ethical ideas—despite the divergence on many matters among thinkers considered here—may help us ground a psychoanalytic conception of empathy.

Let us begin with Plato, who believed that the least tangible things were the most real and most knowable. For Plato, and for such later Platonists as Plotinus, Augustine, and even Aquinas, knowing is a kind of loving participation in the being of the known. Plato portrayed knowledge as generated by Eros:

> The nature of the true lover of knowledge [is] to strive emulously for the true being and . . . he would linger over the many particulars that are opined to be real, but would hold on his way, and the edge of his passion would not be blunted nor would his desire fail till he came into touch with the nature of each thing in itself by that part of his soul to which it belongs to lay hold on that kind of reality—the part akin to it, namely—and through that approaching it, and consorting with reality really, he would beget intelligence and truth, attain to knowledge, and truly live and grow, and so find surcease from his travail of soul. (*Republic,* VI, 490a–b)

Although Plato's view of knowledge may appear unidirectional— the known affects the knower but not the reverse—he did provide clues to the reciprocal nature of empathy. Empathy is a kind of knowledge by contact, contact that depends on kinship and a passion for understanding. For Plato this way of knowing provides access to the fully real. The knowledge emerges from a quasi-erotic contact between the knower and the known, a kind of mutual participation in each other's being. Plato conceived the whole Socratic dialogue as a conversation from which knowledge may arise. For him, even thinking, which he defined as: "a discourse that the mind carries on with itself about any subject it is considering" (*Theatetus,* 189e), is implied conversation. We might view such internal conversation as a precursor to the dialogue that produces empathic understanding.

Aristotle also provided some clues leading to a philosophical conception of empathy. Consistent with his strongly held conviction that we are by nature social and political beings, he provided an account of friendship as a key, if not *the* key, to making a good human being. In loving a friend, Aristotle (*Nichomachean Ethics*) thought, "men love what is good for themselves; for the good man in becoming a friend becomes a good to his friend" (p. 1064). Kohut's (1984) portrayal of the healthy adult as one who is surrounded by empathic selfobjects resonates with Aristotle's emphasis on friendship. Aristotle characterized friends as grieving and rejoicing with one another. In addition, discussion and thought are among the fruits of friendship. And, like Plato, Aristotle regarded conversation as the best way to seek knowledge.

Later, Spinoza (1677) offered an account of knowing that illuminates the concept of empathy. For Spinoza, there were three degrees of knowledge: (1) confused ideas or opinions, or the images of particulars (we might call this common sense); (2) adequate ideas, general and symbolic (our scientific theories); and (3) *scientia intuitiva,* or knowledge of God (or Nature), which leads to an adequate knowledge of the essence of things. This third kind of knowledge is "the intellectual love of God," that is, it is knowledge based on relatedness and on participation in the reality known. Since the knower is part of the reality known (i.e., God/Nature), the knower cannot be outside the reality known, as in scientific empiricism. Likewise, it follows that human beings can know one another only because they are both parts of, or at least participants in, a larger common reality, however we may conceive that larger whole.

In the 20th century, Martin Buber (1937) similarly distinguished between the I-It relation of empiricist observation and manipulation and the I-Thou, or personal, relation. Only in the I-Thou relation is genuine knowledge of another human being possible. As for Spinoza, true knowledge depends on being inside the reality known, or in a relationship encompassing self and other. We perceive, classify, and subdue *things,* such as trees. Nevertheless, if the tree becomes a Thou, it becomes a subject to me, an *other.* Similarly we can treat or describe or classify a human being as an object; only when he or she becomes Thou can there be relation, and true knowledge. In relation to the Thou, I become I.

Empathy is the knowledge that emerges from personal relation and that creates the other as a subject. It is every bit as real and important as—but distinctly different from—the knowledge gained by measuring and counting. "The relation to the Thou is direct. No system of ideas, no foreknowledge, and no fancy intervene between I and Thou" (Buber, 1937, p. 11). Though Spinoza captured the complexity of relatedness more successfully, Buber forces us to recognize that subjectivity becomes real only when two subjectivities meet in a personal relation. Only in such a relation can we empathically know—not just know about—one another. Patients have occasionally remarked that although they know little about me, they feel that they know me very well. Buber would not find such a comment surprising.

American pragmatist Charles Sanders Peirce's view that all reality is continuous (a philosophy he called "synechism") provides another framework for comprehending empathy philosophically. Although he did not discuss in detail the implications of his philosophy of continuity for understanding communication between people, Peirce (1931–1935) did comment that if correct, it would make sense of "the very extraordinary insight which some persons are able to gain into others from indications so slight that it is difficult to ascertain what they are" (vol. 6, par. 161).

Each of the philosophers discussed above views reality as continuous and knowledge as participation in the common reality. Empathy, I believe, is emotional knowledge gained by participation in a shared reality. It is knowledge arising from attunement, to borrow a notion from current infant research. Empathic parents or therapists are those who are attuned to the emotional reality shared in the intersubjective situation (Agosta, 1984). Empathic response comes from attunement to this shared reality, and must take form at a frequency or in a mode (auditory or visual, for example) that the receiver can comprehend. An empathic environment, to which Kohut so often referred, is one in which each person can feel like a Thou, a respected and admired partner in a conversation. Nonresponse or misattuned responses are temporary lapses in empathic understanding.

For Kohut (1981), the most surprising, and almost embarrassing, admission he found himself forced to make about empathy was that it can sometimes heal all by itself. He believed that the fear of death itself could be understood as the fear of the loss of a connection to the empathic, responsive human environment. In support of this view, he cited the case of the astronauts who wanted, if they had to die in space, to at least have their remains return to earth, to the human world. Why should empathy, Kohut wondered, even apart from interpretation, have such fundamental and therapeutic importance for human beings?

To answer this question, we must, with Kohut, view a human being as a social animal whose existence as a self depends on participation in the human world. When people feel completely cut off from empathic response and admiration, they experience disintegration anxiety. Feeling understood and responded to helps a person feel connected to others and thereby safe enough to develop and realize personal aims and ideals.

Empathy in psychoanalysis, nevertheless, or "sustained empathic inquiry" (Stolorow et al., 1987), is no simple matter. It requires substantial attunement to the patient's subjective world, often necessitating a level of consistency captured by the word "sustained." For example, it took me a good deal of time, inquiry, and close observation to understand what my 20-year-old patient meant by telling me he should get a parrot instead of paying to talk with me. Initially, of course, it felt like a simple put-down: Nothing you say is more helpful or intelligent than a tape-recorder or a parrot would be. Gradually we discovered that understanding-sounding words had been used in a disrespectful and intrusive way in his family. Words had described elaborate plans that were never realized, and he had been left with a strong sense of needing a kind of holding that mere words, however understanding, could never provide. As some of these meanings became clearer to us, he became able to ask for a kind of mutual involvement in planning concrete changes in his life, especially in his patterns of self-destructive behavior. Only later did he gradually become more interested in analyzing the meanings.

Empathic understanding includes response.[*] Such response

---

[*]To think otherwise is to lose the pragmatic conception of meaning and return to the isolated mind fallacy (Stolorow & Atwood, 1992). Patients rightly accuse us of not understanding if we do not respond.

may involve words, gestures, practical interventions like adjusting the heat and light for the patient's comfort, or even silence. If a parent knows that a child is being mistreated and does not protect the child, that parent *does not understand* in any practical sense. Thus empathy, including empathic response, is a necessary condition for understanding. In psychoanalytic epistemology, empathy defines the way of knowing—vicarious introspection—and the nature of the known—complex psychological configurations—that we seek to understand in depth. Understanding, as we will see, is a relational and intersubjective conception of psychoanalytic purpose.

PSYCHOANALYTIC UNDERSTANDING

Psychoanalytic understanding is both relational and intersubjective. As a relational reality, the only important concern for psychoanalytic understanding is the human subjective world, or organization of experience. This organized selfhood emerges, continues, and changes only in specific relational contexts. Similarly, it is only when relatedness is present that even partial understanding of the subjective experience of another is possible.

By calling psychoanalytic understanding intersubjective, I mean to draw attention to several of its essential features. First, unlike isolated mind epistemologies, it requires a context of secure attachment, which, in turn, forms the basis of primary selfobject relatedness (Lessem & Orange, 1993). Similarly, the intersubjectivity theory of Stolorow et al. (1987) sees primary emotional bonds as life-giving.* Although some understanding can occur outside important emotional bonds, the capacity for empathic understanding originally takes form, and later develops, in such bonds. The psychoanalytic understanding that heals and promotes emotional growth requires such ties.

Second, intersubjectivity theory best describes the interplay and the shared suffering of psychoanalytic understanding. While this theory recognizes with Sullivan (1953) that "we are all more

---

*They also stress the potentially pathogenic nature of these bonds when their price is the loss or nonformation of organized self-experience.

simply human than otherwise" (p. 32), it also insists that we are "differently organized, interacting subjective worlds" (Stolorow et al., 1987, p. ix). The challenge of understanding arises from the need to recognize, acknowledge, respect, and, at least temporarily, transcend these differences. The dialogue of difference can involve struggle and suffering; in the words of Gadamer, we "undergo the situation" with the other.

Third, intersubjectivity theory, like contemporary semiotics, recognizes understanding as triadic. The triadic nature of understanding means more than your subjectivity, my subjectivity, and our relatedness. It means that yours and mine assume their particular shape in our relatedness. Semiotics (the study of signification) recognizes that all contact between subjectivities requires a mediating sign, a third term. From Peirce (1931–1935) to Umberto Eco (1992), semiotic philosophers have sought to generalize the communicative process of understanding. While they may not use the words *relational* or *intersubjective,* they eschew the isolated mind (Stolorow & Atwood, 1992) and claim that understanding is triadic.

In addition, psychoanalytic intersubjectivity theory as articulated by Stolorow, Brandchaft, and Atwood is a field theory of understanding. Field is a metaphor borrowed from physics. It attempts to address the complexity of causality and influence. Gadamer's metaphor of interplay makes a similar attempt, and it highlights the elements of emergent novelty and surprise. Both metaphors—of field and interplay—transcend the debates about one- or two-person psychologies in favor of a triad of two subjectivities and the emerging understanding that contains and informs them. An intersubjectively oriented supervisor, then, will attempt to evoke descriptions of all elements of the triad: the therapist's subjectivity, the patient's subjectivity, and the emerging and changing sense of the "we."

DEVELOPMENTAL UNDERSTANDING

Psychoanalysis understands developmentally. Every psychoanalytic tradition has emphasized development, and each one has formulated explicit and implicit theories about how development works to form personality. Freud's drive theory and his developmental theories are interrelated. Developmental history is the story of the drives, and interpreting the drives requires a developmental context in which wish, fantasy, and compromise take shape in an individual life. For Ferenczi and his theoretical descendants in Britain and America, knowing the relational history is decisive for understanding how a person becomes a particular self-in-relation. The "complex mental states" Kohut sought to know by vicarious introspection are those of a becoming and historical person. Sullivan, founder of the interpersonalist tradition, wrote detailed and eloquent accounts of the relational development of pathologies. Thus psychoanalysis has always contained a marked "developmental tilt" (Mitchell, 1988). This is so much the case that no one wonders why psychoanalysts, rather than behavioral or cognitive therapists, have been fascinated with recent infant research. Understanding a person psychoanalytically has always included understanding how a particular person developed and who this person is becoming.

So why discuss the developmental nature of psychoanalytic understanding? First, prominent relational theorists have challenged the central focus on development in psychoanalysis, and they have spotlighted instead the here-and-now transference–countertransference interaction. Second, the developmental conception itself needs to be clarified and extended. Third, recent findings in developmental psychology have raised important questions for psychoanalysis, both as a theory and as a set of practices. Finally, I believe that development is the original *what* that psychoanalysis understands and that psychoanalyses (including psychoanalytic therapies) are themselves a developmental second chance.

Several important contributors to the current shift toward a relational psychoanalytic paradigm have challenged the centrality of development in psychoanalytic thought and practice. Prominent among these is Mitchell (1988) whose term "developmental tilt" has become a catchword for those who believe in working primarily or exclusively (Gill, 1982) in the here-and-now, "in the transference." For Mitchell (1988), developmental tilt "collapses relational needs in general into the kinds of interactions which characterize the relationship between the small child and the mother" (p. 152) and "lends a regressive cast to the psychoanalytic enterprise" (p. 152).

Similarly, Greenberg (1992) argues that our adult patients are not children and that we are working with adult minds. In his words, "both our clinical and theoretical goals are best served when we keep in mind that the psychoanalytic situation is an encounter between two grown-up people, negotiating a relationship that will facilitate the ability of one of them to overcome some serious difficulties in living" (p. 285).

Criticism of the focus on development in psychoanalysis has come from those who study countertransference and the influence of the analyst's subjectivity on the psychoanalytic situation. Beginning with Racker (1968), extending through Gill (1982) and Hoffman (1983), and into the work of Ogden (1986, 1989), theorists have seen the analytic situation less as repetition, memory, or reenactment, and more as a relational construction by two people in the present. My response to this argument is that transference and countertransference are themselves developmental and relational ideas. People come into treatment because they can no longer afford to recycle their history; it creates too much pollution in their current lives. Yet unwittingly they repeat their patterns with us—who are full of our own memories and organizing principles—hoping that in a context of understanding they can reprocess what they experience as garbage into something productive. Yes, they are adults, but they feel trapped in the patterns of childhood, and they want to escape these through a new experience with us. This is why I call psychoanalysis a developmental second chance.

A related current of thought is the narrative view of psychoanalysis. It might seem that viewing psychoanalysis as narrative construction would support a developmental view. On close inspection, however, we see that narrative constructivists view the narratives as arising in the here-and-now of the analytic situation, bearing little identifiable connection to the history of either member of the "analytic couple." Instead, the patient's life story is viewed as a product of current conversation. For Spence (1982), unwitting interpretation by the analyst inevitably and perniciously forms the narrative. Similarly, Schafer (1983) believes analysts are always "constructing models of the analysand" (p. 39). Within this view, what the analyst knows empathically is not so much the patient as the model constructed in the analysis. The developmental histories of patient and analyst are peripheral issues.

There are two conceptual issues embedded in the opposition to developmental thinking in psychoanalysis. First, those who ally themselves with this position may fear the emergence of reductive and constricting theories of human nature. For Gerson (1993), any theory of human nature—Daniel Stern's (1985) view of infants' natural capacities and tendencies toward representation of relational experience, for example—is dangerous for psychoanalysis. The danger lies, apparently, not only in the neglect of the infant's family context but also in old or new forms of psychoanalytic realism that may outlast the currently popular skepticism and relativism.* She fears that someone may claim that some features of human nature are given, even universal. Gerson's views, however, are problematic. We must decide these issues on their merits. Not every form of realism is pernicious (Orange, 1992a, 1992b), and some forms of extreme skepticism undermine the healing purpose of psychoanalytic treatment because they discount all paradigms, some of which may have clinical usefulness. Worse, they discount and invalidate patients' experience of their own lives and of their psychoanalytic treatment. We cannot discard every theory of human nature just by calling it a theory of human nature. Developmental theories probably belong in psychoanalysis exactly to the extent that they further understanding, and they deserve exclusion or rethinking to the extent that they restrict or hamper it. Each theory deserves consideration on its own merits.

The other conceptual issue concerns the extent to which eliminating developmental thinking leads to an unintendedly static view of the analytic interaction. Relatedness becomes a snapshot in which two people communicate in a veritable historical vacuum. A view of transference–countertransference relatedness that excludes a developmental perspective misses the texture and process included in an intersubjective approach, in which the two participants bring both a formative history and "developmental strivings" (Fosshage, 1992b). Also, by insisting that knowledge consists of what is observable, the interpersonalists, with their here-and-now focus, inadvertently return to the very positivism that relational theorists generally abhor. Granted, narrative constructivism is not classical positivism, which ignored the influence of the observer

---

*Realism is the philosophical belief that some things are, at least partially, independent of our knowledge or opinions about them. Extreme relativists dispute this claim.

on the observed and on the observing process. It does, however, share the positivist penchant for isolating whatever is observed from its historical context.

Developmental understanding can enrich and inform relational theories of psychoanalysis. In particular, transference and countertransference—or cotransference (Orange, 1994)—can be developmental experiences for both participants in psychoanalysis. They are developmental in at least three senses of the word. First, in transference and countertransference we relive, or emotionally remember, our past relational experience in the present, as the current relationship triggers or evokes either particular memories or more generalized organizations of emotional experience. Second, the relational experience in analysis—no matter what the analyst's opinion about wishes and needs (Shabad, 1993)—is an attempt in the present to repair or restore defective, lost, or traumatic relational experiences (Emde, 1988b). Third, analysis, far from concerning primarily the here-and-now, involves development toward a future. Fosshage (1992b) emphasizes developmental strivings, and Emde (1988b) stresses the influence of the analyst's positive emotions on forward-moving development. Both express the conviction—as held by philosopher Henri Bergson (1910)—that past, present, and future include each other. The future is the least considered dimension of historical and developmental thinking. The realization of the missing dimension of the future leads directly to the need to clarify the conception of development and its place in psychoanalysis.

It is impossible to address the nature of development without considering ideas about truth and reality (explored further in Chapter 10). To develop is to change from something real into something not entirely different. (Patients often find this implicit attitude toward change comforting and encouraging.) The potential for becoming signifies that something had to exist originally. Not that human development, like Aristotle's acorn becoming an oak, is simple and linear. Still, potentials limit outcomes, so we must find out, to the best of our ability, what these real potentials are. Further, as Ferenczi, Balint, Winnicott, Bowlby, Kohut, and other developmentally oriented psychoanalysts have taught us, the relational conditions into which a baby is born limit, catalyze, or even shape potentials.

We can learn little about human potentials or about what relational conditions support their flourishing if we believe we can know nothing, that all truth is construction or fiction (Geha, 1993). We need a pragmatic, fallibilistic conception of good-enough truth. Only then can we converse with other human sciences and allow their thinking to enrich ours and affect our clinical work. Developmental psychologists tell us, for example, that securely attached toddlers become curious and well-related school-age children. As moderate realists, we can then profitably wonder about how these findings bear on our experience in psychoanalytic relationships. If we acknowledge that there is some real difference between more and less adequate human functioning (a moderate claim of a moderate realism), we can search for ever-more-adequate knowledge about what supports and impedes its development. If, conversely, we deny such real differences, we reduce developmental thinking to cultural construction.

A developmental view of psychoanalytic understanding, thus, relies on a moderate realist epistemology, and it works toward ever-more-adequate conceptions of human nature to guide our work and our theorizing. In addition, it implies that there is some substance to the ideas of permanence, change, and continuity through change. These notions may seem abstract, but they are crucial to theories of development and of psychoanalytic cure. Hope for change, at least in feeling states, motivates seekers of treatment. Since change implies temporality, we inevitably face the question of the nature of emotional development, and whether it differs from cognitive forms of change.

Piagetian cognitive development proceeds by assimilation and accommodation. Assimilation strengthens schemata already in place, while accommodation to new experience or to new cognitive capacities modifies them. It might seem that emotional development works in the same way. Assimilation surely occurs, for better or worse. Difficulties with accommodating new experience, that is, with changing the schemata—or emotional convictions—have produced the ubiquitous ideas of resistance (an idea borrowed from physics) and repetition in psychoanalysis. Old organizations of experience stay in place in the face of massive counterevidence. Why? Perhaps psychoanalytic change is not like Piagetian accommodation after all. Psychoanalytic protest against Alexander's program of corrective emotional experience suggests that we have always had doubts about the possibility of transforming what is old.

Perhaps the "new beginning" idea (Balint, 1968; A. Ornstein, 1991) has some merit as an alternative to Piagetian accommodation. Maybe significant change can only occur by making a new start in the emotional life. Stolorow (1994) has begun to think, and I do similarly, that old organizing principles, and old ways of responding and relating, are never eradicated. They remain in place and come alive in stressful situations that replicate old relational and emotional experience. For many of our patients, new relational experience is almost completely new, and it does not fit anywhere in the old organization of experience. Thus psychoanalysis offers a second chance at healthy emotional development in a life that has convinced a person that nothing new is possible. This is the most profound meaning of calling psychoanalytic treatment a developmental kind of understanding.

Let us now consider some important features of developmental understanding. Kohut highlighted the developmental function of mirroring for the creation and maintenance of stable and positive selfhood. His metaphor of the mirror, of the gleam in the parent's eye, however apt and evocative, needs enriching and complexifying. Mirroring involves recognition of something of oneself in the other—Kohut's "chip off the old block" (1977, p. 13). This recognition, in turn, requires an intersubjective conception of mirroring. It implies both particularity and mutuality. I recognize you, and you see that it is you that I recognize. When recognition becomes fully mutual, we recognize each other. Then senses of self, other, and "we" begin to form (Emde, 1988a). When we recognize in one another a common emotional response to something, we enter the developmental stage that Daniel Stern (1985) calls intersubjectivity.

Developmental understanding also establishes or consolidates the sense of one's importance to another. A patient told me that a characterization I voiced about her life meant that I had "considered" her as she had never felt considered. She explained that to say what I had said to her I had to have given serious thought to who she was. She felt that both her parents had been far too self-absorbed to "consider" her. I think much of the therapeutic effect of analytic interpretation may lie, not so much in the insights provided or even jointly found, but instead in the patient's experiencing for the first time being important enough to a parent-substitute to be thoughtfully considered. Conversely, of course, the sense of not being adequately considered by the therapist can lead to rupture or impasse.

Perhaps the most important requirement for emotional development in psychoanalysis is the analyst's emotional availability. Such availability is necessary for participatory knowing, for shared understanding. Whether one considers oneself a Piagetian developmentalist or believes in new beginnings, the analyst's ability and willingness to stay with the patient emotionally provide powerful support for cognitive and emotional growth. Unfortunately, patients often experience interpretation—including developmental interpretation—as our emotional retreat from them. The developmental character of understanding requires that we stay close to the patient's emotional life and reattune as needed. (We will return to the topic of emotional availability in Chapter 9.)

Psychoanalysis is a developmental undertaking in several respects. As a science, it studies human capacities when acute or chronic trauma or deprivation has disrupted healthy growth, and when adaptation to trauma or deprivation continues to disrupt or restrict love, play, and work. As a therapy, psychoanalysis is an opportunity to understand and be understood through a shared emotional experience, to sit *shiveh* together for the child whose early experience cannot be repaired, and to create, through "making sense together," a second chance at developing a good human life. The central and fundamental purpose of psychoanalysis as a therapy, and what distinguishes it from any short-term therapy, is this developmental purpose, this orientation toward the future through the past. A psychoanalysis makes the future possible through a shared experience of one person's past in the present of both people.

Psychoanalytic understanding, then, is the collaborative effort to understand the origins and meanings of a person's emotional life. In the intersubjective field formed by transference and countertransference, patient and analyst come to know by participation in each other's emotional life. This kind of understanding, both process and product, heals because emotional ills require emotional remedies. For many of us humans, the greatest pain and despair come from feeling that our lives and suffering make no sense. Experiencing them as absurd is what makes them unbearable. Making sense together with a trusted guide, especially making sense of one's experience with that guide, can provide something of a "new beginning" in the emotional life.

CHAPTER 3

Theory-Choice
and Fallibilism

> A well-schooled man is one who searches for
> that degree of precision in each kind of study
> which the nature of the subject at hand admits.
> —ARISTOTLE, *Nicomachean Ethics*

*T*he process of understanding has its own requirements. (A philosopher would speak of the "conditions for the possibility of something." A college catalog would say "prerequisites.") To make sense together and to understand emotionally, we need specific intellectual equipment and attitudes. The history of philosophy can provide some clues to what is needed for understanding in general and for that special in-depth emotional understanding that is psychoanalytic.

Philosophers, like psychoanalysts, usually want to go deeper, to examine the assumptions or preconceptions underlying any question. One form of this inquiry is to seek the conditions—necessary or sufficient—for the existence or truth of whatever one is considering. The search for the sufficient conditions for the existence or truth of anything is possible only in either a closed logical system or for the mind of a deity. Since psychoanalysis is neither a closed system nor a deity, we can speak only of necessary conditions for psychoanalytic understanding. These conditions include both intellectual necessities, like theory and an attitude of fallibilism, and practical necessities, like emotional availability and consistency. Undoubtedly others exist. Here let us consider theory and fallibilism; practical necessities will be addressed in later chapters.

THEORY-CHOICE AND RATIONALITY

Psychoanalytic understanding includes both theory and practice. Both theory and practice are forms of understanding. My view of psychoanalytic understanding as primarily clinical, as a collaborative search for a shared web of meanings, does not diminish the need for theory. To guide responsive understanding, psychoanalysis needs conceptual frameworks, complex sets of organizing principles to guide our more reflexive and automatic responses. Theories usually run quietly in the background, ordering the chaos of perception and of the data derived from sustained empathic inquiry. But, if theories are to aid and not impede our work, they often need attention and improvement, sometimes requiring serious rethinking. However, if we choose theories from moment to moment and hour to hour, we risk the integrity and reasonable consistency of our understanding. We thus confront the serious problem of theory-choice.

Analysts today view the theory–practice connection in several ways. Some argue that different theories work better in the hands of individual practitioners. Others, such as Pine (1990), believe that different theories work better with specific sorts of patients. According to this view, a good analyst, like an accomplished violinist who can play Bach, Mozart, or Brahms as the program requires, has a flexible repertoire of practical interventions based on theories of drive, ego, object, and self. Yet others assert that over time there has been some convergence and some consensus; some "common ground" has emerged (Wallerstein, 1992). Freudians protest that they are no longer so distant and silent as relational analysts portray them. Alternatively, Mitchell (1988, 1993) argues that many schools of psychoanalytic theory and practice have made a fundamental shift to a relational model, with its interest in mutuality and presence.

Still, many issues remain hotly debated and most analysts

maintain an identification with the school of thought in which they were trained. Two issues of the journal *Psychoanalytic Inquiry* (Pulver, Escoll, & Fischer, 1987; J. Miller & Post, 1990) studied the shaping of practice by theory, and they exposed profound continuing differences in the ways psychoanalysts allying themselves with different theories speak with patients in daily clinical work. In each issue a prominent analyst provided clinical material, including transcripts of taped sessions. Analysts from various schools of thought were invited to comment. The differences in the ways analysts thought they would respond struck this reader as significant, which suggests that our choice of theory may seriously affect the ways in which we work with patients.

On what grounds do we choose our theories? Granted, people develop and hold theories that express their subjective organizations of experience (Atwood & Stolorow, 1993). This observation points us toward a study of the personal and inter-subjective dialogic processes involved in the making of theory. Here, however, I consider a different question. What are reasonable grounds for preferring one theory to another? Although we may no longer find the scientific rationality that shaped the Freudian enterprise useful (Mitchell, 1993), many of us revise our theories during our professional lives on what we think are reasonable grounds. Freud himself, for example, was in part a pragmatist who revised his theories as he stumbled on new clinical evidence. He was less concerned with consistency in theory—he explicitly denied any interest in philosophy—than with finding some explanation for the phenomena he observed. Likewise Kohut saw new clinical findings as reasonable grounds for theory-revision. This sense of "reasonable grounds" expresses an often unarticulated commitment to a particular conception of reasonableness. I will therefore briefly outline some history of reasonable grounds and reasonableness so we can see how they bear on theory-choice in psychoanalysis.

The history of philosophy demonstrates that the question of reasonableness arises in various ways, each of which focuses on a particular form of the problem: What is reason? What is it to think rationally? When does a person think or act reasonably? How does reason differ from what is not reason, that is, from the irrational and the nonrational? These formulations of the question, scarcely the only versions, are not strictly equivalent. Yet each is a part of our question about reasonable grounds for theory-choice and theory-improvement. Restricting the consideration to one form of the question would impoverish the inquiry. So, at the risk of probably unavoidable ambiguities, let us approach each philosophy in the following discussion through its own way of posing the question, keeping in mind our question of reasonable grounds for theory-choice.

PHILOSOPHY AND REASONABLENESS

In the world of myth prior to the advent of philosophy, each event required a single explanation, usually the arbitrary will of an anthropomorphic deity. The pre-Socratic philosophers of the fourth and fifth centuries B.C.E. (Kirk & Raven, 1984) sought, for the first time, a consistent account of *reasons* "behind" events, *reasons* underlying the patterns they found in nature. Thus, a change in their experience took place: They no longer perceived each event as a single, or unique, phenomenon, but as part of some generality. Parmenides and Heraclitus, commonly seen as antagonists, both sought this "generality" in whatever continues through change. Parmenides distinguished the way of truth from the way of seeming or appearance. He thought reasonableness consisted in recognizing that truth is more than appearance. He made a major step toward a conception of reason that somehow penetrates beyond the appearance of what we see with our eyes. For Parmenides, attention to what changes without recognition of persistent structure, or *logos,* was not reasonable.

Although Heraclitus emphasized change over permanence, he too drew attention to a *logos* ruling the world. To hold, as Heraclitus did, that everything changes, is not to say that all change is random. Thus Heraclitus attempted, even more than Parmenides perhaps, to account for permanence of patterns in the experienced world. Further, both Parmenides and Heraclitus wanted, each in his own way, to view the world as a whole. Insisting on generality, they thus developed the first complex description of reasonableness in the Western tradition. In Parmenides and Heraclitus we already find intimations of criteria for theory-choice: Reason concerns more than fleeting appearances and is related to what is general and what endures.

By the time of the atomists, Epicureans, and Stoics, the search for generality had turned toward the ethical. The ancients had begun to search for patterns of life that would lead to human satisfaction. Their first problem was to identify the nature of such satisfaction. To Democritus, for example, the highest good was a mind without fear. The next step was to discover how to order human conduct to promote such aims. Rationality now meant adapting means to ends, fitting patterns of action to theories of the good. These thinkers pointed toward pragmatic criteria for the rationality of theory-choice.

By far the most important advance came, of course, with Socrates, Plato, and Aristotle. Socrates, as Plato portrayed him, embodied reasonableness. Socrates had no answers, no theories, only an insatiable thirst for understanding, for making sense. Yet for Plato himself, to think or act was to proceed according to general reason, to participate in a Form,* and to know that one is doing so. Although he accorded a prominent place to myth in his dialogues, Plato did not retreat from his project of rationality. Instead he recognized that reason includes much of what the search for it can lead to denying—such elements as intuition, myth, and a search for beauty and truth. We can know the Form of the Good only by a flash of insight (*Letter VII*, 341c). Still, he did contrast reason with opinion, which he understood as receiving one's views primarily from the crowd. Although Plato affirmed the necessary relation of rationality to an objective universal beyond the knower, he recognized that rationality can be only the rationality appropriated by a knower. He would have recognized the common clinical finding that emotional reorganization, a "new beginning," is necessary to make insight curative. Only reasonableness that one can emotionally own makes a difference.

With Aristotle came the first system of formal logic and the first formal attention to reason itself. Aristotle was confident both that the cosmos—including human life—is intelligible and that human beings can understand it. Further, he identified the contemplative

---

*For Plato (*Republic*, VII), only the Forms, or Ideas, were fully real. What most of us consider real are mere shadows or reflections which have only a shared, or derivative, reality and cannot truly be known.

or theoretical life of reason itself as the highest human good. To Aristotle we also owe the distinction between practical and theoretical reason. For him, practical–productive knowing has its source in the knower and in the knower's purposes. *Theoria,* on the contrary, is thinking for which the source, principle, or origin is in the object known, not in the scientist. Ethics and politics represent the practical; physics is an example of theoretical science. (It is probably safe to assume that Aristotle would have seen psychology and psychoanalysis as parts of practical reason, since they concern the good human life.) However, even for Aristotle who saw them as distinct, the practical and the theoretical are closely interwoven. In Aristotle's *Nicomachean Ethics,* the application of theory became the ultimate motivation for all the practical sciences. For both Plato and Aristotle, rationality is a quality more of wise people than of theories. The best theory is the one that a wise person would choose.

In modern philosophy, Kant (1929) offered a "critique of pure reason," arguing that such reason is insufficient to inform us about anything. For Kant, to be reasonable is to decide carefully the limits of the knowable and to conduct inquiries inside those limits, in constant acknowledgment of those limits. Reason is a cautious affair of seeking in human life the meaning and direction of human life. For Kant, theory exists for the sake of practice. Theoretical entities— God, freedom, and the immortality of the soul—are conditions for the possibility of the practical moral life. Even physics, he thought, involves elements of such practical values and interests. Kant treated philosophy as a project of limiting idle speculation, and he pointed out the practical interest inherent in all reason. He also directed us to pragmatic consequence as a criterion for theory-choice. His ethical "categorical imperative"—act as if the principle of your action should become a law of nature—affirmed the centrality of generalizability as a rule for theory-choice. An excessively particular theory, or one we would not want applied to ourselves, is excluded by the Kantian view of rationality or reasonableness.

For Hegel, on the contrary, reason meant seeing any event as part of a larger whole, especially seeing it historically. To reason is not to subject reason itself to a Kantian critique, but instead to place ideas and events in context, especially in temporal context. Hegel (1807) called the organizer of experience a "subject": "Reason appeals to the self-consciousness of any and every subject " (p.

275). True objectivity, for Hegel, meant recognition of the rule of rational subjectivity, "self-conscious reason" (Lauer, 1976, p. 11). Theory, for a Hegelian, requires reference to subjectivity, to the dialectic, and always to history.*

American philosopher Charles Sanders Peirce (d. 1914) gave the question of rationality, or in his words "reasonableness," a pragmatic form. His conception of rational purpose, or concrete reasonableness, overcame the dichotomy between theoretical and practical reason, and it provided guidance for theory-choice. Habit, he believed, is generality in purposeful action or thought. Reason is the power to form or change habit by reflection on experience. Reasoning itself is thinking according to habit, to be subjected to the same critical review as other habits. Peirce recognized that theory-choice has personal and subjective elements. Still, any such choice implies a claim of reasonableness transcending idiosyncrasy. Kant's view of morality had required generality—take as your moral maxim what you want applied to every case. Similarly, the "categorical imperative," or fundamental moral duty, for Peirce is to *think* so that the maxim, or logical organizing principle, of one's reasoning can extend consistently to all thinking.

Peirce's concrete reasonableness (cf. Orange, 1984), however, is partly an ideal; it does not already exist fully as an absolute measure of theories. Since our yardstick is only emerging, we thus must always be cautious, Peirce thought, about calling the enterprises of others irrational. As far as they are products of human purpose, the things that others do are rational in part. They are efforts to order means to ends, and to promote the emergence of truth. To aim for the *summum bonum* (the ultimate good), or concrete reasonableness, requires Peirce's community of inquirers, whose categorical imperative is to promote reasonableness. The growth of reasonableness, for Peirce, is the most satisfactory ideal aim of all practice. We might add that contributing to the development of reasonable psychoanalytic theory is one reasonable aim of psychoanalytic practice.

---

*The Hegelian roots of intersubjectivity theory may be minimized for fear of the tyranny of teleology, the assumption that process has some kind of inherent, predetermined outcome. There is no Absolute Spirit in intersubjective theory. We could argue, however, that Hegel's teleology differs from Aristotle's simple acorn becoming an oak. Just as in evolution, development need not mean the outcome is predetermined.

In our century Alfred North Whitehead (1938) both clarified and undermined the distinction between speculative and practical reason. In his view, the speculative reason of Plato seeks complete understanding, whereas practical reason, the rationality of Ulysses, seeks immediate methods of action. Speculative reason and practical reason are, however, only forms of reason; each, for Whitehead, is incomplete and dangerous without the other. "Some of the major disasters of mankind have been produced by the narrowness of men with a good methodology. Ulysses has no use for Plato, and the bones of his companions are strewn on many a reef and many an isle" (p. 12). (Warnings against "wild analysis" contain this caution about practice without theory.) A Whiteheadian would insist that theory-choice is crucial, but that it involves a continuing interchange between the speculative and the practical.

Yet holding theory in any reasonable way requires thought, evaluation, and choice. Philosopher Robert Nozick (1993), in *The Nature of Rationality*, suggests two rules for theory-choice, or rational belief: "not believing any statement less credible than some incompatible alternative—the intellectual component—but then believing a statement only if the expected utility (or decision-value) of doing so is greater than that of not believing it—the practical component" (p. xiv). Since Nozick shares the pragmatists' conception of belief as that on which one is prepared to act, his criteria depend on what he means by "credible" and "utility." He understands credibility as consisting of cognitive qualities like coherence and plausibility. Utility includes emotional qualities. Rationality, therefore, means the making of both cognitive and emotional sense. Any proposal for belief that falls short of both deserves skepticism.

REASONABLE CRITERIA FOR
THEORY-CHOICE IN PSYCHOANALYSIS

What makes it more reasonable to hold one theory than another? Using the ideas of the philosophers discussed above, and referring to the discussion of understanding in Chapter 2, I think we can establish several important criteria: inclusiveness or universalizability, practical bearings, and coherence.

Plato, Hegel, and Peirce would all unite to reject scientific positivism and reductionism in favor of inclusiveness. Similarly, some criticisms of drive theory in psychoanalysis treat inclusiveness as a criterion. According to this argument, human motivation and experience include attachment, artistic creativity, interests in self-development, scientific curiosity, spirituality, and, especially, the organization of experience. A theory that reduces away major realms of human experience should be rejected in favor of a more inclusive theory. Lichtenberg's (1989) work on motivational systems grounded in developmental psychology, is a serious attempt at greater inclusiveness in psychoanalytic theory. Kohut and others have made a similar argument about analyzability. If psychoanalysis claims to contain universal truth and wisdom about human beings, but then finds most of those who seek it too ill for psychoanalytic treatment, something must be wrong with the theory. Those who embrace object relations and self psychological approaches to treatment have claimed that their theories apply more universally.

Consideration of inclusiveness leads us directly to the question of practical bearings, a second criterion for theory-choice in psychoanalysis. When good-enough theory is used, it makes a practical difference. Granted, each school of thought claims its theory, well applied, yields better results in more cases than other theories do. My point is that *effects are reasonable grounds for theory-choice.* In psychoanalysis particularly, we have a constant personal and professional interest in continuing to develop theories that work well. We thus aim to prevent the rigidification of theory. Stolorow (1988) has formulated a set of questions that captures the intellectual and practical issues involved in theory-choice:

(1) Does a psychoanalytic framework permit greater inclusiveness and generality than previous ones: Does it encompass domains of experience mapped separately by earlier, competing theories, so that an enlarged and more unified perspective becomes possible? (2) Is the framework self-reflexive and self-corrective? Does the theory include *itself* in the empirical domain to be explained? (3) Most important, does the framework significantly enhance our capacity to gain empathic access to subjective worlds in all their richness and diversity? (pp. 336–337)

I suspect much variation in theory occurs because each theory positions the analyst differently vis-à-vis the patient in the intersubjective field. With different theories in mind, analysts attend to different elements in the psychoanalytic field, and in turn their different responses create different events to observe. These differences become evident as we listen to discussions of psychoanalytic neutrality and intimacy. The classical analyst is the out-of-sight observer who takes no position in the disputes among id, ego, and superego (A. Freud, 1936). The object relations analyst, "without memory and without desire" (Bion, 1967), maintains a similar neutrality among the patient's internal objects. An interpersonalist sits emotionally across from the patient, like a friendly opponent and teacher in chess or tennis. The self psychologist, unabashedly partial to the patient, sits on the patient's side, helping the patient sort out the inner chaos from within the patient's perspective and develop a strong self.*

These positional differences suggest that psychoanalytic theories involve ways of being with people. Analysts attempt to arrange the intersubjective field according to their theories and organizing principles for the presumed benefit of the patient and for their own emotional comfort. Theoretical progress may depend on the emergence of a consensus about the relative efficacy of these ways of being relational. Yet analysts will always vary in comfort with various forms of intimacy, and consensus may prove elusive. What works best for one analyst may not be reasonable—in the sense of practical reason—for another.

The third consideration for theory-choice is coherence: Everyone—even the most committed empiricist—wants a coherent theory. Those who consider themselves correspondence theorists—for whom truth is a match between thing and idea, original and copy—still shudder at charges of intellectual incoherence. If our opinions seem inconsistent, most of us feel an almost moral obligation to find ways to harmonize them. Thus eclectic attempts to hold several theories whose underlying assumptions are incompatible are generally unsatisfying. It may also be because of this discomfort that some theories favor reductionistic explanations.

---

*Fosshage (1992a) suggests that we shift back and forth between two of these positions or attitudes: outside (the interpersonalist's position) and within (the self psychologist's attitude) the patient's perspective

They do reduce incoherence. However, for those who squirm in the confines of reductionism, the challenge lies in framing more inclusive theories or paradigms (Kuhn, 1962). These must account for the diversity of phenomena so that all the theoretical assumptions and available data fit together. I believe a reasonable psychoanalysis can settle for no less demanding an ideal of rationality.

Seeing theories as Peircean (1931–1935) "habits of belief" may help to demonstrate the importance of theory-choice. Habits can be good, bad, and better. They can change when human purposes change. They can be more or less reasonable, not only by formal logical criteria but also insofar as they meet the demands of generality and conduce toward short-term and ultimate human goals. In psychoanalysis, of course, these goals include healing through psychoanalytic understanding. *If the primary goal of psychoanalysis is the reorganization of a person's experiential world, a reasonable theory will lead us toward this end.* Unfortunately, progress toward such an end is difficult to measure. This complication leads us to consider some forms of uncertainty involved in psychoanalysis.

UNDERSTANDING AND NOT KNOWING, OR PSYCHOANALYTIC FALLIBILISM

A second necessity for any reasonable psychoanalytic epistemology is fallibilism, an attitude recognizing that what we "know" or understand is inevitably partial and often mistaken. The word "fallibilism"' emerged in the philosophy of science as a reaction against the Roman Catholic declaration of papal infallibility. According to this doctrine, the pope cannot be wrong when he speaks *ex cathedra* (from the papal chair) on matters of faith or morals. Philosophers like Peirce contrasted the attitude of science—"contrite fallibilism"—with what they saw as the complete dogmatism and irrationalism of organized religion.

However, the desire to know that we know is not restricted to religion. A student recently asked me how to know when we have reached truth or understanding in clinical work. My answer included reference to pragmatic criteria: to effects on the patient's life and good-enough understanding within the psychoanalytic process. I also mentioned the Socratic view that wisdom often consists in recognizing that we do not know.

My student's question, however, contains an assumption derived from the epistemological inquiries of modern philosophy, namely, that we need to be certain that we know (Bernstein, 1983, calls this "Cartesian anxiety"). Many philosophers of this century have emphatically abandoned the search for certainty as the index of truth. Both American and continental thinkers have appealed to logic, the philosophy of science, evolutionary biology, human psychological experience, and Heisenberg's uncertainty principle to support their contention that reality evolves and that the knower inevitably affects the known. Theories themselves undergo both gradual transformation—as they are explored in the community of inquirers (Peirce, 1931-1935)—and replacement (Kuhn, 1962). Yet psychoanalytic writings and curricula often express, if only indirectly, the view that a received body of truth about human psychological functioning—metapsychology—and about the process of change in this functioning—clinical theory—already exists. In this view, we may need only to refine theory and to apply it more skillfully; nevertheless, the core of truth is already available.

The Critique of Positivism within Philosophy

American philosophers—in this respect returning to the ancient Socratic ideal—have refocused our attention on the process of inquiry. Peirce (1877) described in "The Fixation of Belief" methods people use to remove "the irritation of doubt" to settle their beliefs. Having dismissed the methods of tenacity and authority, he described the method of science. Peirce, like Kuhn a century later, was thinking of the physical sciences, the Copernican and Darwinian revolutions. For Peirce, science is a public and self-correcting method by which a surprising fact evokes a hypothesis for testing. If it survives, we hold it as theory only until the next surprising fact comes along. Belief, then, is the absence of actual, practical doubt. In psychoanalysis, such surprising facts leading to theory-revision have included Freud's discovery of transference and Ferenczi's recognition of the prevalence of child abuse. Today the discovery of extensive cognitive–relational capacities and interactional processes in infancy may be surprising facts leading to new beliefs.

Peirce often cautioned, however, that we must hold beliefs lightly so we can notice surprising facts and keep the process of inquiry self-corrective. As an antidote to dogmatism, he suggested that there should be a large sign at the front of every classroom that reads: "Do not block the path of inquiry." The ultimate outcome of inquiry, the truth, according to Peirce, would be the opinion reached "in the long run" by the community of inquirers. (More recently, Kohut, 1973, urged that psychoanalysts think and function in the community of scholars.)

Peirce's friend William James (1907) spoke of the "cash value" of ideas and truth as what "works." By his provocative expressions he meant to draw attention to his "radical empiricism" (p. 6). He thought that all matters for philosophical reflection and inquiry are questions drawn from experience and are ultimately resolvable by an appeal to experience. Truth, for James (1909), consisted of a continual structured process of exchange and of checking between ideas and experience: "Truth *happens* to an idea. . . . It *becomes* true, is *made* true by events" (p. 3). Not that an idea is untrue until experience confirms it; the idea is just pragmatically and experientially empty.

More recently, American historians and philosophers of science—Kuhn and Popper, for example—have drawn attention to the process character of truth and of the search for truth in the scientific community. Kuhn (1962) describes the replacement of important theories, or of overarching paradigms, by more inclusive theories, as well as the immense resistance new ideas generally meet.* He attributes this resistance to the intrinsic character of normal science with its organizational structure and processes— journals, curricula, tenure, and conferences. These, he thinks, can impede the dissemination, nurturance, and adoption of new ideas. Popper (1959), in another vein, saw the holding of assumptions not in principle or practice falsifiable as a major impediment to growth and change in scientific theory.

---

*I recently heard a story, perhaps apocryphal, that British psychoanalyst Susan Isaacs returned home distressed from a psychoanalytic meeting at which her thoughts had been treated harshly. Her allergist husband is said to have commented, "There is no more powerful allergen than a new idea."

Popper (1959), in another vein, saw the holding of assumptions not in principle or practice falsifiable as a major impediment to growth and change in scientific theory.

Similarly, continental thinkers like Husserl (1931) have advocated a return from dogma to experience. Husserl advocated the method of transcendental phenomenology, the bracketing or holding in abeyance (epochē) of all preconceptions to achieve pure experience and to know the essence of ideas. Today most psychologists and philosophers agree that all experience—even perception—is structured, that observation is theory-laden, and that Husserlian presuppositionless knowing is impossible. Still, Husserl's exhortation has further encouraged both the "holding lightly" of theories and a close attention to experience.

Philosophical hermeneutics has added force to the rejection of the search for certainty, particularly in the human sciences. Hermeneutics calls into question the assumption that questions of meaning ever have just one correct answer (Palmer, 1969). Hermeneutics, at least agnostic on the question of ultimate truth, attempts to explore the multifaceted interpretations of biblical texts, of literary works, and, increasingly, of human experiences. It not only questions the search for a single correct interpretation but it also replaces the objectivist approach to the text or to the experiencing human being. Instead we have phenomenological inquiry aware of itself as affecting and being affected by the text or the feeling person. Quantum physics had found that the fundamental characteristics of the physical world were affected by attempts to measure them. Similarly, hermeneutics rejects the objectivist assumptions underlying much "scientific" thinking. Instead it has embraced a focus on subjectivity and intersubjectivity, thereby requiring us to replace the search for certainty with an acceptance of the fallibility of knowledge.

The Critique of Positivism within Psychoanalysis

Freud envisioned psychoanalysis as a science in the spirit of 19th-century positivism, modeled on biological neuroscience (Sulloway, 1979). The empirical methods of psychoanalysis, he

---

[*] Ellenberger (1970) notes that the young Freud spent a year translating into German works of English empiricist John Stuart Mill into German.

origin and holding power to the Freudian hope that the pure data—the patient's associations—could be examined in an uncontaminated form on a "blank screen" so that correct interpretations and reliable theories would result.

Since the middle of this century many psychoanalysts have challenged this view of the psychoanalyst as anonymous and detached researcher delivering correct interpretations. Like Ferenczi, who cared more for therapeutic efficacy than for Freud's ideal of scientific purity, some analysts have suggested more engagement with the patient. Citing the vast differences in patients' presenting difficulties, Alexander and French (1946) urged a much greater than customary flexibility in practice. They proposed that psychoanalysis be defined less by its technical rules and by the development of a transference neurosis. Instead, they thought that psychoanalysis is defined by its basis in psychodynamic principles and by its goals. While Alexander has been largely associated with the notion of "corrective emotional experience," his primary concern was for attention to the individual patient's needs and for the abandonment of rigidity. Precisely because people are individuals, Alexander believed, psychoanalysis must be an inherently uncertain and tentative enterprise. Alexander's "flexibility" paid close attention to the patient's idiosyncratic ways of making sense of experience. Alexander's approach presages the "optimal responsiveness" Bacal (1985) suggests as a replacement for abstinence and frustration. Flexibility and responsiveness based on empathic understanding are incompatible with a rigid investment in correctness or certainty.

George Klein (1976) suggested that the superstructure of metapsychology had obstructed our capacity to learn from clinical data. He attempted a "theorectomy" on Freud's work. He wanted to sift out the clinically rich suggestions from what he saw as the needless Procrustean bed of experience-distant theories of motivation and personality that have become known as psychoanalytic theory. Partly inspired by Klein's work, I here note the continued attachment of analysts to such Procrustean beds, both in theory and in practice, and I will suggest a possible explanation for such continued attachment.

Like Klein, Atwood and Stolorow (1984) have made a radical departure—similar to Kant's "subjective turn" in the history of philosophy. They avoid rigid *a priori* notions of personality and motivation. Their "psychoanalytic phenomenology" explicitly eschews rigid adherence to drive theory or to tripartite psychic structures. Instead they advocate a focus on the subjective organization of the patient's experience of self and other. They urge the formulation of descriptions of pathology, motivation, and the therapeutic process in experience-near terms. To explain how the analyst hears, they replace the expectations drawn from metapsychology with the personal organizing activity of analyst and patient.

With their psychoanalytic intersubjectivity theory, Stolorow, Brandchaft, and Atwood (1987) carry this approach a step further. They focus on the intersubjective character of the mutual search for understanding—not for certainty or absolutes—in psychoanalysis. Like quantum physicists who found that the knower affects the known even in physics, they insist that the organization of the patient's subjective experience is intelligible only as it has taken form in an intersubjective context. This view depends on—although the authors do not make this explicit—a process philosophy of knowledge and reality similar to that articulated by Alfred North Whitehead (1929), who held that every "actual entity" continually *creates itself in relation* with other actual entities by selectively including and excluding facets of these other entities. To state the obvious, *no one comes into being alone.* Such a relational ontology of organic process requires recognition of the continuous participation by both subjects in a psychoanalysis. Both take part in making sense of and in the transformation of subjective worlds.

The Search for Certainty in Contemporary Psychoanalysis

Today we see increasing willingness to hold theories lightly in many quarters (cf. Cooper, 1993). Still, many psychoanalysts remain engaged in a search for certain and reliable answers to questions of theory and technique. This is particularly evident when psychoanalysts attempt to define psychoanalysis. Some discussants seem particularly interested in distinguishing psychoanalysis from psychotherapy. Psychoanalysis, they often claim, includes a belief in unconscious mental processes and a focus in treatment on resistance and transference. Others claim that it is not such theoretical notions that distinguish psychoanalysis from psychotherapy, but rather it is the use of the couch or the frequency of sessions. Others claim that the use of the empathic–introspective method of understanding the subjective world of the patient is the crucial identifying characteristic of psychoanalytic work. William James might have asked us what is the "cash value," or practical bearing, of this discussion.

Discussions of analyzability also seem to reflect a need for certainty. Psychologists attempting to gain admission to a prestigious medical psychoanalytic institute have met suggestions that perhaps they were not "analyzable" and thus not qualified for psychoanalytic training. In addition, some institutes accept the work of candidates only if their patients meet criteria for analyzability. Such distinctions seem primarily to serve the maintenance of power and control, to rationalize treatment failures, and to preserve the self-respect of those who make them. More flexible thinking has led to the search for theories and methods that would regard more people as analyzable. Many are also considering the possibility that analyzability resides in the analytic couple, not in the individual.

Another example of the search for single right answers is the quest for the "correct" interpretation. Interpretations may seem correct because they emerge from the assumptions of a familiar psychoanalytic theory. Like some scientific theories, they may be simple, parsimonious, and "elegant." On more pragmatic grounds, they may yield more associations by the patient. Surely some interpretations—usually those that come more from antecedently held theories by the analyst than from close attention to the patient—can be harmful. What remains puzzling is the importance placed on a kind of objective correctness instead of on a mutual engagement in coming to understand or in a healing process. This phenomenon suggests that analysts may at times be more invested in seeking a kind of cognitive truth—which provides us a feeling of being grounded somewhere—than in understanding emotional chaos with its messy fringes.

Practical questions, often raised by candidates in psychoanalytic institutes and answered by senior analysts, and sometimes even discussed in psychoanalytic conferences and journals, carry an urgency that bespeaks a need for Cartesian "clear and distinct ideas." Ought I ever to reveal my experience to the patient? Must every patient use the couch? Is any action besides verbal interchange acceptable in a psychoanalysis? Such earnest questions suggest an assumption that learning psychoanalysis requires finding generally applicable answers to such procedural questions.

The urgency of the questions may also reflect the felt threat to our self-cohesion that some patients evoke. Kohut (1984) gave an example of the rigidity that results from the analyst's need to follow rules of technique:

> I know of one analysis, for example, which, after making steady progress with a severely traumatized patient for two years, came to grief because the analyst insisted on changing the position of her chair in order to prevent her patient from continuing to glance at her face at certain crucial moments. The analyst tried to justify this move to the analysand by telling him that the rules of analysis prohibited this kind of gratification—that gratifying him by making her emotionally involved face available to him would be an obstacle to "remembering" and "working through." She thereby repeated the chronically cold attitude of the patient's schizoid mother who had imposed bizarre rules of behavior on the child from the time he was born and had been unable to respond to him with natural warmth and concern. The analysand felt unable to tolerate this change and ended treatment. (p. 220)

This example illustrates an adherence to rigid procedural rules, rationalized as necessary for the patient's cure, but applied without reference to the patient's experience. Apparently such rigidity supported the analyst's positive evaluation of herself as a professional. Kohut's story also demonstrates the disastrous results of such rigidity and provides a clue to the possible causes of many treatment failures. Of course, transferential responses will emerge in response to other analytic attitudes or patterns—for example, unusual flexibility may be experienced as retraumatization by a patient whose parents were grossly inconsistent, perhaps alcoholic. Here, however, our concern is with the harmful effects of rules intended to support the analyst's search for certainty.

Historically, the institutionalism reflected in such concerns for correctness in theory and technique may have originated in Freud's separation from official medicine and the resulting need to give psychoanalysts a physician-like status. Freud's concern to protect the reputation of his psychoanalytic movement was another source of analytic reliance on rules (Ricci & Broucek, 1994). Ellenberger (1970) notes that "With Freud begins the era of the newer dynamic schools, with their official doctrine, their rigid organization, their specialized journals, their closed membership, and the prolonged initiation imposed upon their members" (p. 418).

Why does the search for certainty and correctness in theory and in practice persist among psychoanalysts? I believe that this search concretely expresses analysts' needs for selfobject experiences (Bacal & Thomson, 1993) to maintain a stable psychological organization in the face of the chaos and pain we meet continually in our work. Without correct theories, correct interpretations, and correct techniques to rely on in our many moments of doubt, we might lose hold of our selves. We might feel afraid or fragmented. Old pain and confusion might rise to haunt our work. I think that much of the rigidity and the search for correctness detailed above is an attempt to protect us from these frightening threats to our organized sense of stable self-experience.

The Fallibilist Alternative

With other sorts of support for the practitioner—peer groups, supervision, satisfying personal ties, and absorbing outside interests—the questions and concerns might change, and uncertainty might become less anxiety-provoding. We might ask what kinds of interventions, interpretations, and responses promote mutual understanding of the patient's organization of experience? How are emotional ties between patients and therapists established, maintained, and restored? What is the relationship between these bonds and the process of change? How can we learn from our failures or mistakes? In other words, holding our theories lightly—both general and clinical theories—will not only require that we seek support for our personal stability elsewhere. It may also enable us, both individually and collectively, to continue theory development in creative directions that we might never see if we continue the search for certainty to maintain the stability of our organization of experience. Theories that recognize the fallible nature of all understanding might also reduce some of our shame over not knowing. In other words, our shame and anxiety can give way to a liberating Peircean "contrite fallibilism."

To summarize, in this chapter I have argued for two intellectual conditions for the possibility of good-enough analytic work, which are also two necessary elements of any adequate psychoanalytic epistemology. First, we need theory, carefully chosen according to some ideal of reasonableness. The refusal of theory-choice is the refusal to think through and organize our analytic experience on both sides of the room or the couch. This refusal is a choice of relativism, a return to Hegel's "night in which all cows are black." Second, we must hold our theories lightly, in a fallibilistic spirit, ready to be surprised and prepared to admit our theoretical and clinical mistakes. Analytic training should prepare candidates to think, not just to absorb the theories of others, and to revise their thinking as needed.

In later chapters I will consider some practical and emotional conditions for the possibility of good-enough psychoanalytic understanding.

CHAPTER 4

Toward an Epistemology of Perspectival Realism

"*I* am so confused," patients tell me almost daily. They refer to emotional bewilderment and disorientation, the sources and implications of which we seek to understand. Making sense together often helps to clear the muddy waters. In the same collaborative spirit, we psychoanalytic colleagues can approach conceptual confusions that interfere with our professional communication and our theorizing.

The process of understanding, psychoanalytic and otherwise, often envolves embracing ambiguity but attempting to clear up confusion. Ambiguity and confusion differ. Ambiguity occurs when a term has more than one common meaning, and a speaker or writer either chooses not to, or fails to, specify the intended meaning. Sometimes, as recognized by the psychoanalytic principles of multiple function and overdetermination, removing ambiguity results in oversimplification. Often we must simply live with ambiguity. Conceptual confusion, on the other hand, most often results when speakers or writers do not know the common denotation or connotation of a term, or how to distinguish it from related words. Sometimes both ambiguity and confusion appear today in contemporary discussions by psychoanalysts of the philosophical questions crucial to our profession's self-understanding. While the ambiguities may be harmless, the confusions can place us in a clinical fog, unable to help our patients find a good-enough sense of reality because we do not know how to find one for ourselves. To clear up the confusion, we need careful distinctions.

Philosophers have long made distinctions their stock in trade. In that tradition, I attempt here a modest and limited task: to draw three distinctions and to point out their importance for psychoanalytic theory. Specifically, I distinguish between subjectivity and subjectivism, between subjectivism and relativism, and between objectivism and realism. These distinctions will allow me to articulate the epistemology that I believe is fitting to describe psychoanalytic understanding as an intersubjective process. I call this view "perspectival realism."

SUBJECTIVITY VERSUS SUBJECTIVISM

In current usage, the term "subjectivity" roughly replaces Freud's concept of "psychic reality." However, the equivalence is not precise because "psychic reality" implies the existence or significance of "external reality" while "subjectivity," most commonly referring to the personal organization of experience, leaves open the question of external or objective reality. Atwood and Stolorow (1984) borrow the term subjectivity from Husserl's transcendental phenomenology. They enrich it with the views expressed in Kohut's seminal paper, "Introspection, Empathy, and Psychoanalysis" (1959), in which he claimed unequivocally that the domain of psychoanalysis is limited to whatever is accessible through introspection and empathy. Subjectivity includes both process, the activity of organizing experience, and product, the organization of experience, which is understood as a relatively enduring configuration. This enduring *Gestalt* shapes and limits a person's future experience and activity.

Subjectivity differs from subjectivism. Epistemological subjectivism holds the Cartesian view that truth and knowledge are accessible only via individual subjectivity. Ethical subjectivism means that the goodness or evil of actions depends on the subject's view of them, that moral values are radically individual. Epistemological subjectivism, as, for example, embraced by Husserl but not by all those inspired by his transcendental phenomenology, ends in radical solipsism. In solipsism the knowable is merely the content of one's own mind. For Atwood and Stolorow (1984), "The practice of transcendental phenomenology presents a spectacle of thought detached from social life, circling inwardly upon itself and mistaking a reified symbol of its own solitude for the discovery of its absolute foundation" (p. 13). Husserl's phenomenology insists on the universality of the reduction, or "epochē"—taking nothing for granted. It recognizes as valid only what originates in subjectivity. In the words of historian of phenomenology Herbert Spiegelberg (1960):

> While it is true that Husserl is the founder and remains the central figure of the [phenomenological] movement he is also its most radical representative and that not only in the sense that he tried to go to the roots, but that he kept digging deeper and deeper, often undermining his own earlier results; he was always the most extreme member of his movement, and hence became increasingly the loneliest of them all. (p. xviii)

In Lauer's (1978) words, the phenomenological project ends with only "Edmund Husserl himself in splendid isolation" (p. 165).

Nevertheless, just as phenomenology extends beyond Husserl's own view, the emphasis on the study of subjectivity inspired by Husserl is not coextensive with Husserl's subjectivism/solipsism. As Lauer (1978) notes, "there can be no question that, historically speaking, phenomenology has in recent times performed the important philosophical function of directing attention more seriously to experience as the only legitimate starting point of philosophizing" (p. 167). Similarly, we might say that phenomenology has pointed psychoanalysis toward its only legitimate starting point, the subject's experience. Any phenomenological view of the method and theory of psychoanalysis (Kohut, 1959; Atwood & Stolorow, 1984) requires that we put aside preconceptions—diagnostic, metapsychological, and otherwise—to work as completely as possible within the subjective experience of the patient. Only by placing our theoretical and other preconceptions aside can we gain insight into the essential structures of the patient's subjectivity. The qualifier "as possible" recognizes the limits on this phenomenological project that are imposed by our own historically constituted subjectivity, our organization of experience. Although Husserl, who did not concern himself with understanding others' experience, took little interest in these limits, we cannot avoid them. Sometimes we recognize them under the rubric of "countertransference," or what an intersubjectivity theorist might name cotransference (see Chapter 5 for distinction between countertransference and cotransference). In addition, we now know that we must recognize our inevitable influence on the patient's subjective experience.

For Husserl (1931), however, the search for the essential structures of subjectivity has to precede any consideration of the phenomena of intersubjectivity, and this belief prevented his philosophy from ever getting to an exploration of intersubjectivity's properties and implications. The radically ahistorical character of Husserl's phenomenology prevented the consideration of the effects of past relational experience on a person's subjectivity. Similarly, the complete suspension of preconceptions eliminated relational patterns from the search for present structures of subjectivity. Psychoanalytic phenomenology—in order to be psychoanalytic—must take our past and present experience of others into account. It must thus be less philosophically radical than Husserl was. We can leave to philosophers the task of deciding whether a phenomenology embedded in history and relatedness is still phenomenology. My point is that defining the domain of psychoanalysis as the domain of the subjective organization of experience need not commit us to the radical subjectivism or solipsism of Husserl. Instead we give our subjectivity essence and structure by assimilating and organizing past and present experience, especially relational experience. I know myself as a tenacious or disciplined person, for example, by making sense of the responses of others to my work habits. Such experiential knowledge contains both what is given—my weed-pulling, house-painting, or writing—and my subjective organization of the given within intersubjective fields.

SUBJECTIVISM VERSUS RELATIVISM

Subjectivism is not coextensive with relativism and may not even be compatible with it. Relativism, an approach that views knowledge as radically dependent on theory, social context, circumstance, or utility, denies the existence of any universal truth or moral framework. Truth, for the relativist, varies with socially constructed theoretical frameworks and is not, as for the subjectivist, a product of the individual's subjectivity. Goldberg (1988), for example, views relativism as a denial of objectivism: "Relativism is a viewpoint that considers the world as a variable thing that need have no inherent composition save as we choose to categorize it" (p. 44). A relativist can evaluate truth or morality only from within a socially agreed-upon system. For a moral relativist, situational criteria external to the moral agent decide the morality of particular actions. A subjectivist, on the contrary, understands morality as a function of the individual's preferences or values. Both subjectivists and relativists deny the existence of universal truths or moral values. However, where they locate the truths and moral criteria they do recognize differs widely: The subjectivist places them in the individual, the relativist in the theoretical framework or social context. American philosopher Richard Bernstein (1983) carefully distinguishes subjectivism from relativism. In his view, an absolute subjectivist like Husserl was no relativist. His transcendental phenomenology was "intended to be the definitive answer to all forms of relativism, skepticism, and historicism" (p. 11). Conversely, a relativist may not be a subjectivist. In Bernstein's words:

> His or her [the relativist's] essential claim is that there can be no higher appeal than to a given conceptual scheme, language game, set of social practices, or historical epoch. There is a nonreducible plurality of such schemes, paradigms, and practices; there is no substantive overarching framework in which radically different and alternative schemes are commensurable—no universal standard that somehow stands outside of and above these competing alternatives. But the relativist does not necessarily claim that there is anything subjective about these schemes, paradigms, and practices. (pp. 11–12)

We might reasonably ask Bernstein whether a relativist could *ever* be a subjectivist. Relativism here appears not as Husserlian subjectivism but as a Protagorean epistemology and as a moral position rejecting universals. Protagoras's "man is the measure" does not mean that individual subjectivity is the ultimate reality or the moral court of last appeal. Protagorean relativism means, as Bernstein says, that "there can be no higher appeal than to a given conceptual scheme, language game, set of social practices, or historical epoch." It is perhaps this meaning that Fosshage (1994) intends when he contrasts relativism with scientific positivism, suggesting that relativism makes better sense of the psychoanalytic situation and especially of the forms of relatedness we call transference and countertransference. Still, relativism continues to be vulnerable to the traditional charge of incoherence: To compare relativism and positivism, one must take a nonrelativistic epistemological position that can in turn be evaluated from another external position, and so on to infinite regress. One must take a nonrelativistic position to choose relativism. Indeed, one must be a nonrelativist even to choose among theories. Psychoanalysis, therefore, needs alternatives to relativism, as well as positivism, scientific empiricism, and naive realism. It is precisely this need that my third distinction will address.

OBJECTIVISM VERSUS REALISM

Distinguishing subjectivism from relativism prepares us to consider so-called objective reality and its bearing on the psychoanalytic concentration on experience. An exclusive focus on the experiential world of the patient may appear to neglect what interpersonalists call "problems in living." Empathic introspection, or sustained empathic inquiry, may seem to restrict, even to eliminate, the analyst's access to data available through normal perceptual processes. As European thinkers like Gadamer and Habermas might ask, What good is a world of meanings detached from praxis, the action that proceeds from practical wisdom?

To avoid the conceptual problems inherent in subjectivism and in self-contradictory relativism, and to avoid the neglect of practical realities, we need to distinguish between objectivism and realism (cf. Potter, 1994). The exact definitions and history of various objectivisms need not concern us here. What they have in common—in contrast to all forms of subjectivism and relativism—is the claim that there are fundamental and universal criteria for judging truth and falsehood, right and wrong. A common form of objectivism, also known as empiricism, holds that the ultimate court of appeal is something called "objective reality," or "the facts." In midcentury philosophy of science (Hempel, 1951; Popper, 1959), this empiricism demanded that any theory, to qualify as scientific, had to meet the test of falsifiability. That is, the proponents of the theory had to specify what experimental results would lead to the rejection or falsification of the theory. The human sciences (*Geisteswissenschaften*), including psychoanalysis, could thus be easily excluded from the true sciences, along with religion, metaphysics, and astrology. Only a theory open to falsification by experimental evidence could be called scientific or had any "cognitive significance" (Hempel, 1951; Suppe, 1977). In this spirit, psychoanalytic objectivists have viewed transference as distortion that can be seen by the observer/analyst to be distortion when compared with the facts, and they regard the capacity for access to the facts, or good reality-testing, as a major criterion of psychological health.

Postempiricist philosophy of science, as represented by Kuhn, Feyerabend, Hesse, and others, has almost universally rejected the form of empiricist epistemology that demands falsifiability. British philosopher Mary Hesse (1980) usefully attacks the underlying assumption that radical differences exist between the natural sciences and the human sciences. She details five contrasts thought by objectivists to divide the natural and the human sciences. The first and fifth of these supposed contrasts are most salient for the point of view I am advocating:

> 1. In natural science experience is taken to be objective, testable, and independent of theoretical explanation. In human science data are not detachable from theory, for what count as data are determined in the light of some theoretical interpretation, and the facts themselves have to be reconstructed in the light of interpretation. . . .
>
> 5. Meanings in natural science are separate from facts. Meanings in human science are what constitute facts, for data consist of documents, inscriptions, intentional behaviour, social rules, human artifacts, and the like, and these are inseparable from their meanings for agents. (pp. 170–171)

Suppose these differences between the natural and human sciences truly existed. Then transference would resemble mere human science, a distortion or even a delusion when compared with the objectively verifiable facts provided by the natural sciences, evidence provided by medical tests, say. Yet every characteristic of the human sciences listed above is now assigned to the natural sciences as well. Thus current philosophy of science challenges such venerable psychoanalytic conceptions as transference-as-distortion and reality-testing. Hesse goes on to summarize the conclusions of postempiricist philosophies of science that undermine the contrasts:

> 1. In natural science data [are] not detachable from theory, for what count as data are determined in the light of some theoretical interpretation, and the facts themselves have to be reconstructed in the light of interpretation. . . .
> 5. Meanings in natural science are determined by theory; they are understood by theoretical coherence rather than by correspondence with facts. (pp. 171–172)

Rejecting these contrasts does not mean there are no differences between the natural and the human sciences. Nevertheless, their differences do not consist in an honorific scientific status accorded to so-called objective facts. The empiricism so soundly rejected in recent philosophy of science remains, however, popular in psychoanalysis (Hanly, 1992). Our theory and practice have remained relatively insulated from, and, until the recent past, unaffected by university-based ferment in the philosophy of science. Since Freud's time, psychoanalysis has a long tradition of calling itself a science and of wishing to be a natural science in that honorific and empiricist sense. Perhaps, in addition, working wholly in the realm of meanings leads psychoanalysts to yearn for the certainty and apparent security of facts and universals. Anyway, postempiricist understandings of the nature of science make considerable room for forms of psychoanalysis that avoid an allegiance to objective reality, especially those that embrace intersubjectivity and other relational theories.

The rejection of objectivism does not imply the falsehood of every form of philosophical realism. Realism is the view that some matters do not depend on our opinions about them. A realist believes there is something, or at least something emerging, to be more fully known, discovered, or articulated. In the words of Peirce (1868), "The real . . . is that which, sooner or later, information and reasoning would finally result in, and is which is therefore independent of the vagaries of me and you" (p. 168). Peirce thereby provided a thoroughgoing process conception of reality.*

Scientific empiricism, which we should be careful not to equate with science, is a popular modern version of objectivist commonsense realism, with its associated assumption that observer and observed are independent of each other. Its Popperian form requires that proponents of any theory specify those factual conditions that would lead them to consider the theory inadequate—the falsifiability criterion. Even in the natural sciences, such empiricist realism has been out of date since the emergence of quantum physics, with its insistence on the impact of the observer on whatever is to be observed. Correspondence theories of truth, according to which truth consists in a match between things and the ideas that are thought to be copies of them, now seem naive.

Other forms of realism, especially those that see truth as gradually emergent in a community of inquirers (Peirce, 1931–1935), or in a dialogic community, show more promise. One version of this communitarian or intersubjective (Bernstein, 1992) realism might be a perspectivalism that would conceive of reality as socially understood or as a socially articulated process. Each participant in the inquiry has a perspective that gives access to a part or an aspect of reality. An infinite—or at least an indefinite—number of such perspectives is possible. (Hoffman, 1983, applies a similar perspectivalism to transference and countertransference.) Since none of us can entirely escape the confines of our personal perspective, our view of truth is necessarily partial, but conversation can increase our access to the whole.

Such an intersubjective–perspectivalist realism—what I am calling perspectival realism—is not equivalent to the cultural and epistemological relativism mentioned earlier. Instead, cultures and

---

*Ironically the original philosophical meaning of realism (i.e., that universals exist apart from human knowledge of them) originated with Plato, who eschewed every form of commonsense realism.

theories themselves are perspectives on emergent truth. Nor does such realism describe the historical narrative negotiated in treatment (Spence, 1982; Schafer, 1983). Though such negotiation provides a small-scale approximation of the larger process, it can only provide another perspective on "the truth." Instead, perspectival realism recognizes that the only truth or reality to which psychoanalysis provides access is the subjective organization of experience understood in an intersubjective context (Stolorow et al., 1987). Simultaneously, such a subjective organization of experience is one perspective on a larger reality. We never fully attain or know this reality, but we continually approach, apprehend, articulate, and participate in it. In other words, unlike Husserl's phenomenology, an intersubjective theory can admit the importance of social life and of the continuing effect of practical life in the world. Kohut's self psychology views subjectivity as the entire domain of psychoanalysis and sees so-called external events as bearing meaning only as the patient experiences and organizes them. While this view does exclude common-sense realisms, correspondence theories of truth, and scientific empiricisms, it does not exclude the possibility of dialogic, communitarian, or perspectival realism. In such a moderate realism, the real is an emergent, self-correcting process only partly accessible via personal subjectivity but increasingly understandable in communitarian dialogue.

CHAPTER 5

Cotransference: The Analyst's Perspective

Every word is a prejudice.
—Friedrich Nietzsche,
The Wanderer and His Shadow

I grew up as the eldest of 10 children. Everything was scarce, both economically and emotionally. Thus I was raised to be a provider, not a recipient, of care and to value myself primarily for the sheer number of tasks I could do to keep the family going. My earliest memories involve folding diapers and feeling that I was held responsible for allowing any harm to, or misbehavior by, my younger siblings. This history–and much more that I will not detail here–concretely shapes my experience as a clinician. Along with my intellectual and clinical training, this history filters, informs, and organizes both my perception and my responsiveness to patients, whether they be oldest, youngest, middle, or only children.

Psychoanalytic understanding, grounded in intersubjectivity theory, thus, must take into account the analyst's subjective world, including theory, personality, emotional history, and prereflective organizing principles. "Cotransference" primarily names the analyst's contribution to the intersubjective field in psychoanalytic treatment. More broadly, the term refers to the concurrent and mutual organizing activity of analyst and patient. It does not include the traditional reference to distortion or to the correspond-

63

ing idea of an objective reality to which one party has access and the other does not. As a perspectivalist term, it does include the original conception of transfer, or carry-over, from the relational history in which any personal perspective has been formed.

COUNTERTRANSFERENCE IN THE DEVELOPMENT OF SELF PSYCHOLOGY

I begin by examining the concept of countertransference in the development of self psychology. My colleagues from relational perspectives other than self psychology say that self psychology pays too little attention to countertransference. Their helpful critique provoked me into reconsidering the concept of countertransference, and that has led me to develop a concept more consistent with both self psychology and intersubjectivity theory.

Kohut (1971) began his revolutionary *The Analysis of the Self*: "The subject matter of this monograph is the study of certain transference or transferencelike phenomena in the psychoanalysis of narcissistic personalities, and of the analyst's reactions to them, including his countertransferences" (p. 1). By countertransference, Kohut meant remnants of the analyst's own narcissistic disturbances that interfered with the development of and the analysis of the selfobject transferences. He cited, for example, "the tendency of some analysts (at times due to a mobilization of their countertransference) to respond with erroneous or premature or otherwise faulty interpretations when they are idealized by their patients" (p. 138). If such countertransferences are stable, according to Kohut, they often consist of "quasi-theoretical convictions or of specific character defenses or (as is frequently the case) of both" (p. 263). In the final chapters of *The Analysis of the Self*, Kohut devoted considerable attention to countertransferential responses of analysts to the various narcissistic transferences.

Kohut (1984) returned to the topic of countertransference briefly in his posthumous *How Does Analysis Cure?* where he continued to regard it as harmful by definition. "If we want to see clearly," Kohut wrote, "we must keep the lenses of our magnifying glasses clean; we must, in particular, recognize our countertransferences and thus minimize the influence of factors that distort our perception of the analysand's communications and of his personality" (p. 37). He went on to deny the applicability of the influence-of-the-observer-on-the-observed principle in psychoanalysis. Kohut attributed difficulties in analytic understanding to the analyst's "shortcomings as an observing instrument" (p. 38).

Since Kohut saw countertransference as problematic, it may be difficult for self psychologists to view it as an essential part of the theory and process of psychoanalytic cure. In addition, Kohut (1971) thought a good psychoanalytic theory, like a good analytic treatment, should be unrelated to the analyst's personality (pp. 222n–223n). Analysis should be a nonidiosyncratic science that can be taught to noncharismatic practitioners. The practitioners are not, however, to be traditionally neutral. Sustained listening to understand and explain, he thought, is not a neutral activity. I think that Kohut was torn between a desire to emphasize the human determinants in psychoanalysis and his classical training, which, even in his last years, made him want to sift out the personal elements. This ambivalence may have prevented him from conceptualizing countertransference as later self psychologists have.

Wolf (1988), for example, adopts Gill's (1982) usage and sees countertransference more inclusively as the analyst's experience of the relationship (Wolf, 1988, p. 137). He distinguishes among countertransferences, identifying (1) the analyst's pleasure in effectiveness; (2) the "countertransferences proper," which are "based on the analyst's residual archaic selfobject needs" (p. 144); and (3) reactive countertransferences, the tendencies, identified by Kohut, to unmask defensively the idealizing, mirroring, and merger transferences. Since Wolf was one of Kohut's closest collaborators, his move toward an inclusive conceptualization of countertransference is important.

Intersubjectivity theory goes even further toward broadening the meaning of countertransference. For Atwood and Stolorow (1984), the psychoanalytic process emerges from the intersection and interplay of two differently organized subjectivities. In their words, "Patient and analyst together form an indissoluble psychological system" (p. 64). Their vision of psychoanalysis is reminiscent of Gadamer's (1976) account of playful exchange:

> When one enters into dialogue with another person and then is carried along further by the dialogue, it is no longer the will of the individual person, holding itself back or exposing itself, that is determinative. Rather, the law of the subject matter [*die Sache*] is at issue in the dialogue and elicits statement and counterstatement and in the end plays them into each other. (p. 66)

Within such a dialogue, Stolorow et al. (1987) understand countertransference as "a manifestation of the analyst's psychological structures and organizing activity" (Stolorow & Lachmann, 1987, p. 42). They hold that "transference and countertransference together form an intersubjective system of reciprocal mutual influence" (p. 42).

Some self psychologists, especially those influenced by intersubjectivity theory, have thus departed significantly from Kohut's negative view of countertransference, moving toward a more inclusive definition of the word. Self psychology now, even more clearly than before, recognizes the influence of the analyst/observer (whose experience of the analytic relation is countertransference in the inclusive sense) on the observed. Increasingly we find discussions of the analyst's organizing activity, history, and personality in self psychological case reports. We write less often as if the analytic patient were the only one organizing or reorganizing experience (Goldberg, 1988; Thomson, 1991).

However, self psychologists at times can be so involved in and devoted to getting and staying close to the patient's experience that we may forget that we are there too. Thus, our cherished effort to understand our patients from their vantage point may prevent us from recognizing and remembering our contribution to *shaping* the patient's experience (the influence of the observer on the observed). It may also interfere with our seeing that we can understand another's experience only through our own equally subjective experience. In the words of Lomas (1987):

> By the very nature of things people cannot attain perfect openness to each other. Our perceptions are based on past experience. Nothing is entirely new to us, otherwise we would completely fail to appreciate it. However much we strive towards an unencumbered, receptive state of mind, we bring to each exchange the sum total of our history, an interpretation that is unique to us, the most coherent,

manageable and least anguished *Gestalt* that we have been able to attain. (pp. 39–40)

The apparently spreading opposition to viewing transference as distortion is consistent with the acknowledgment that two subjectivities are always at work. Consistency requires that this opposition should expand to eliminate the distortion idea from countertransference.

In addition, I think that the concept of countertransference makes little sense to clinicians who do not subscribe to theories of innate aggression. Self psychologists generally view anger and hostility as understandable responses to deprivation, abuse, and the frustration of crucial emotional needs for appreciation, affirmation, validation, and consistent support. "Counter" suggests, among other things, reacting against, or opposing. This is not comfortable language for psychoanalysts who embrace a relational approach, especially self psychologists, because we usually view ourselves as allied with the patient. At the very least, the traditional use of the term "countertransference" suggests the possibility of standing apart from the patient's experience, as if countertransference were a bounded thing a clinician could *use.* On the contrary, I think understanding is incompatible with standing apart. I believe that the term "cotransference" better conveys our participation *with* the patient in the intersubjective field or play space of the psychoanalytic conversation. This inclusive term removes the connotation that the analytic relation is automatically or in most respects adversarial. Instead it affirms Loewald's (1986) view that

> it is ill-advised, indeed impossible, to treat transference and countertransference as separate issues. They are the two faces of the same dynamic, rooted in the inextricable intertwinings with others in which individual life originates and remains throughout the life of the individual in numberless elaborations, derivatives, and transformations. (p. 276)

"Cotransference" treats the organizing activity of patient and analyst as "two faces of the same dynamic." Neither activity needs a label with pejorative connotations.

"Cotransference," like the related terms "intersubjectivity" and "mutual influence," does not mean that no differences exist between the participation of analysts and that of patients in analysis. To acknowledge, as the cotransference notion does, that psychoanalysis fully involves two subjectivities does not eliminate the important differences between them. The analyst or therapist is always there primarily for the sake of the other. Aron (1992) helpfully articulates this apparent paradox by distinguishing between mutuality and symmetry. Mutuality means, as Eleanor Roosevelt liked to say, that "understanding is a two-way street," that the subjective worlds of both patient and analyst are fully implicated in the process. Symmetry connotes equality, or at least a balance, in the contributions and roles of both partners. Psychoanalysis, in Aron's view and in mine, is a mutual and asymmetrical relationship.

COTRANSFERENCE, EMPATHY, AND HERMENEUTIC INQUIRY

Empathy has occupied a pivotal place in the theory of self psychology because Kohut (1959) insisted that the psychoanalytic realm was by definition coextensive with whatever introspection and empathy (or vicarious introspection) could reveal. Empathy, however, is the knowing activity of a subject who has her or his own psychological organization. Therefore, self psychology especially requires an inclusive notion of countertransference (or cotransference) as a necessary, though not sufficient, condition for the possibility of empathy. By empathy Kohut meant the focused attempt to enter another's subjective reality. Stolorow et al. (1987) call this process "decentering," by which they mean that the therapist may need to expand or modify her own organizing principles in order to understand the patient's subjectivity. A dialogic or perspectival realism requires such vicarious introspection for the communication and sharing of perspectives. Such empathic dialogue may produce both an understanding of already existing perspectives and the creation of new ones. To achieve empathic understanding, I widen my perspective (I do not abandon it) by asking myself how the other person's point of view, feelings, convictions, and responses could make sense, could be reasonable. Because of the need to widen one's perspective to accomodate that of another, empathy is an inherently intersubjective process.*

Philosophical hermeneutics can elucidate the inevitability of cotransference. Hermeneutics, as we have seen, was originally a set of rules or methods for interpreting biblical texts. More recently Schleiermacher and Dilthey identified hermeneutic inquiry as an attempt to read the meaning of a text by reference to the author's intentions (*mens auctoris*). How to gain access to the author's intentions was a practical problem. With the growth of historical consciousness in the past century, hermeneutics has come to include history—we might say development—as vital to understanding anything. Modern hermeneutics has come to view a text or a painting or a dream as a "*Sache selbst*," a thing itself (not just a product of the author's intentions), partly understandable from the perspective of an interpreter. The interpreter participates in a conversation with the text. From this exchange new meanings are always emerging. We can know nothing of the text without knowing the interpreter, including the interpreter's theories, personal history, and organizing principles. There is no single, completely existing truth about the text, person, or dream. Instead, for a hermeneutic thinker, an indefinite number of possible interpreters and perspectives exists. Communication among interpreters with various perspectives may make possible more inclusive and coherent—and in this sense truer—views, perspectives, understandings, and theories.

Gadamer is now the most prominent proponent of hermeneutic perspectivalism. To adopt this view would require a more inclusive psychoanalytic notion of countertransference, or cotransference. Gadamer claims, first, that prejudice is inevitable. By prejudice he means the inescapable being-somewhere vis-à-vis whatever we seek to know or understand. He thus intends to strip "prejudice" of its negative connotations—as difficult a task as

---

*Both within and outside self psychology, there are those who insist that self psychology is a "one-body," not a relational, theory. I believe self psychology's relentless reliance on empathic understanding, an inherently two (or more)-person process, places it clearly among the relational theories in psychoanalysis.

making "countertransference" a neutral or positively valenced term. Here is Gadamer's (1976) attempt:

> It is not so much our judgment [about truth or value] as our prejudices, that constitute our being. This is a provocative formulation, for I am using it to restore to its rightful place a positive concept of prejudice that was driven out of linguistic usage by the French and the English Enlightenment. It can be shown that the concept of prejudice did not originally have the meaning we have attached to it. Prejudices are not necessarily unjustified and erroneous, so that they inevitably distort the truth. In fact, the historicity of our own existence entails that prejudices, in the literal sense of the word, constitute the initial directedness of our whole ability to experience. Prejudices are biases of our openness to the world. They are simply conditions whereby we experience something—whereby what we encounter says something to us. This formulation certainly does not mean that we are enclosed within a wall of prejudices and only let through the narrow portals those things that can produce a pass saying, "Nothing new will be said here." Instead we welcome just that guest who promises something new to our curiosity. (p. 9)

Similarly, American philosopher Peirce (1931–1935) cautioned:

> We cannot begin with complete doubt [in the style of Descartes]. We must begin with all the prejudices which we actually have when we enter upon the study of philosophy. The prejudices are not to be dispelled by a maxim, for they are things which does not occur to us *can* be questioned. (vol. 5, par. 156)

Another way to speak of the necessity of prejudice (or of cotransference) is to consider both the interpretation and the interpreter, and in particular, the historicity of the interpreter. For Gadamer, interpretation is not an attempt to read an author's mind, as Schleiermacher and Dilthey believed. Instead the dialogic process, the interplay of interpreter and text or patient, creates something new: the understanding. Interpreter and text are equally important, and the historicity, including the prejudices (organizing principles), of the interpreter takes on an organizing role. For Gadamer, attributing subjectivity to the text and objectivity to the interpreter dangerously denies the interpreter's contribution to the making of meaning.*

However, I am not advocating that we should simply accept our prejudices or organizing principles; instead we must continually test them. We test them, not by empiricist criteria to check for distortion, but in conversation. Continental philosophers often use the notion of horizon to mean the field of vision, or whatever perspective is available from where one stands. We test our prejudices by attempting to see whether they fit with broadening horizons. Similarly, we may revise our organizing principles (as in Piagetian accommodation) or we may develop new organizing principles (as in a new beginning) to take new experience into account. Colloquially, we sometimes speak of education or travel as "broadening our horizons," enlarging our perspective on the world. Rightly or wrongly, people commonly make the assumption that a broader perspective is likely to be truer and that narrowness is somehow wrongheaded. "Deeper is better" is the psychoanalytic version of that assumption. (To the objection that delusional people claim to see broadly and deeply into meanings, a response might be that we are speaking here of the elaboration of complexity, whereas delusions usually oversimplify.) In the hermeneutical view, we attain a broader or deeper experience of anything first by knowing and acknowledging who we are—our historicity and our prejudices. Only then can we enter the playful exchange that broadens and deepens our understanding.

In psychoanalytic language, we must know and acknowledge our cotransference, our point of view or perspective, if we are to become capable of empathy (or vicarious introspection). In order to do authentic psychoanalytic work, or to speak authentically of our work, we must acknowledge the lenses through which we are reading the text or the patient.

Such a hermeneutical awareness does not address questions

---

*Owen Renik (1993), commenting on the work of Schwaber (1992) has recently expressed this well:

> Instead of saying that it is *difficult* for an analyst to *maintain* a position in which his or her analytic activity objectively focuses on a patient's inner reality, I would say that it is *impossible* for an analyst to be in that position *even for an instant;* since we are constantly acting in the analytic situation on the basis of personal motivations of which we cannot be aware until after the fact, our technique, listening included, is *inescapably subjective.* (p. 560)

about the advisability or inadvisability of so-called countertransference disclosures. Answers to these questions fall within the domain of optimal responsiveness (Bacal, 1985). Normally I decide such matters on pragmatic grounds. Often I must decide quickly, as when a patient asks, "What are you thinking?" or "How do you feel about that?" Sometimes, I honestly have to say that I do not know or cannot quite put it into words yet. The patient thus learns that I too struggle to understand. William James (1902) sometimes formulated the central pragmatic maxim as: "By their fruits shall ye know them" (p. 20). In this view, if a type of intervention or response to a particular patient usually yields understanding and self-consolidation, then it deserves serious consideration, and vice versa.

Under discussion here, instead, is the nature of understanding itself. At issue is the thesis that *cotransference* (or countertransference in the inclusive sense) *is a necessary though not sufficient condition for the possibility of empathy.* Cotransference includes both historicity and the prejudices/horizons of philosophical hermeneutics, which are roughly equivalent to personal history and organizing principles. To understand psychoanalytically, and to understand psychoanalytic understanding, we must acknowledge our personal historicity and examine our prejudices. To work psychoanalytically, we must have access to our historicity. In my case, for example, I need to know how my family position influences my response to only or younger children, whom I may envy, feel excessively responsible for, or see as irresponsible and spoiled. We must also prepare ourselves to criticize our horizons— especially our theories of human nature embedded in our psychoanalytic theories—and to revise those prejudices that limit our capacity to understand another's experience.

Finally, to reexamine the question of the place of countertransference in any psychoanalytic theory, let us turn to the old question of the hermeneutical circle. Many have tried to articulate the paradox that understanding is inevitably circular, that we look to the part to see the whole and to the whole to comprehend the part. Palmer (1969) summarizes the view of early Romantic philologist Friedrich Ast (d. 1841): "Because *Geist* is the source of all development and all becoming, the imprint of the spirit of the whole (*Geist des Ganzen*) is found in the individual part; the part is understood from the whole and the whole from the inner harmony of its parts" (p. 77). Similarly, for Schleiermacher, the whole of the text and the parts of the text explain one another (Palmer, 1969). Dilthey (1989) provides the example of a sentence that can only be understood by grasping the inevitable interaction of the whole and the parts.

This view of understanding has implications for the debate between those who favor here-and-now focus and those who emphasize history and development in clinical work. Neglect of either, in Dilthey's view, would hamper understanding. For our purposes here, however, Dilthey (1989) illuminates the necessity of the dialectic of whole and part, past and present, for understanding. Among Gadamer's (1991) important contributions is that he added the future as a factor in the dialectic. His work demonstrates that the hermeneutic circle is no longer vicious once the historicity and horizons of the interpreter take their rightful place.

Gadamer sees clearly that risking and testing prejudices in "dialogical encounter" is the path to understanding through the hermeneutical circle. The nature of understanding is that alone we can come to understand only what we already understand. To risk testing our organizing principles in dialogue with a text or a person makes possible a new meaning. Such new meaning may be a newly complexified organizing principle or a future form of emotional experience that could emerge only through the conversation. This account of the process of psychoanalytic understanding in the language of intersubjectivity theory (Stolorow et al., 1987) is completely incompatible with objectivist and empiricist theories of truth or with an exclusive psychoanalytic focus on the subjectivity of the patient. Vicarious introspection, or empathy, is implicit conversation between perspectives.

Gadamer's view thus avoids the feared subjectivism and solipsism of the hermeneutical circle. He believes that the path to understanding in the hermeneutical circle runs inevitably through the self-knowledge of the interpreter. If for Gadamer's (1979) "text" we read "patient" and for "understand" we read "empathically understand," the implications for psychoanalytic self psychology, and for any psychoanalytic understanding, become clear:

> In reading a text, in wishing to understand it, what we always expect is that it will *inform* us of something. A consciousness formed by the

authentic hermeneutical attitude will be receptive to the origins and entirely foreign features of that which comes to it from outside its own horizons. Yet this receptivity is not acquired with an objectivist "neutrality": it is neither possible, necessary, nor desirable that we put ourselves within brackets. The hermeneutical attitude supposes only that we self-consciously designate our opinions and prejudices and qualify them as such, and in so doing strip them of their extreme character. In keeping to this attitude we grant the text the opportunity to appear as an authentically different being and to manifest its own truth, over and against our own preconceived notions. (pp. 151–152)

To summarize, I use a perspective derived from philosophical hermeneutics to explain my claim that countertransference in the inclusive sense is indispensable to empathy, that it is a necessary condition for empathy. This conceptualization of countertransference should find a prominent place in self psychology or in any psychoanalytic approach that recognizes empathy as an intersubjective way of knowing. I further suggest that countertransference in this inclusive sense be renamed "cotransference" and that we reserve the term countertransference for the analyst's delimited and reactive emotional memories that interfere with empathic understanding and optimal responsiveness.

CHAPTER 6

Experience: Given and Made

*I*f asked 50 years ago what they seek to understand psychoanalytically, most analysts would have responded either "transference and resistance" or "character." Today we are more likely to say that we seek to understand the experience of another person or, perhaps, the shared experience of the "analytic couple" (Nissim-Momigliano & Robutti, 1992). Nevertheless, we, like our philosophic forebears, may be hard-pressed to say what we mean by "experience." In ordinary speech, people talk of learning from experience or something really being an experience, an event worth remembering. We call someone an "experienced analyst" or an "experienced plumber," and we use "experience" as an active, transitive verb, as in "I experienced that as an insult." Self psychologists claim to stay close to the patient's experience and to theorize in "experience-near" language. The term is slippery and difficult, for reasons that will become evident as we examine its history. Still, a close look at the term and idea "experience" may illuminate, if not resolve, some running debates in psychoanalytic theory. A moderate perspectival realism, or hermeneutic pragmatism, can help us affirm and recognize both the given (brute, unavoidable) and the made (organized, construed) aspects of experiencing. Let us first examine some explicit and implicit conceptions of experience in analytic theorizing.

EXPERIENCE IN PSYCHOANALYTIC THEORY

"Experience" has not traditionally been considered a psychoanalytic term. It does not appear either in the index to the *Standard Edition* of Freud's works or in Moore and Fine's (1990) *Psychoanalytic Terms and Concepts.* Perhaps we take for granted a shared understanding of this term. Nevertheless, radically varied notions of experience underlie and buttress psychoanalytic theories and practices. I will characterize these conceptions as scientific realisms, contemporary idealisms, and mixed conceptions. Later I will return to the philosophical history of the idea of experience.

Scientific realism is the ontological view that what is true and real is actually out there. Accompanying this view is the epistemological claim that we, or at least some of us, can tell what is true and what is false. Such realism is usually tied to a correspondence theory of truth (cf. Protter, 1985; Potter, 1994). Correspondence theory holds that truth consists in a match between already existing facts and our ideas about or words for them. Freud betrayed his scientific realism—including an allegiance to correspondence theory—in his frequent references to "external reality." External reality makes demands on us, disillusions us, deprives us of loved ones, and so on. Nevertheless, it is always something out there, outside the subject, outside psychic reality, irreducibly *given.* When the word "experience" does appear in the *Standard Edition* of Freud's works, it is usually a translation of *Erlebnis,* or experience in the sense of occurrence or event. This usage of the word experience suggests externality largely independent of the subject. The empiricist epistemological project of the scientific realist becomes to decide how, to what extent, and with what degree of certainty, the mind can know the independent reality of the given. The observer has little or no effect on the observed.

American ego psychology emphasized adaptation and reality-testing. It accepted or adopted a correspondence theory of truth (Hanly, 1992) with the associated idea of experience as the more or less accurate registering of what actually happened. The notion of patients distorting and of analysis as correcting these distortions reflects this point of view. Ego psychologists view adaptation to reality as an important component of mental health.

On the other end of the spectrum we find contemporary voices who vociferously oppose scientific realism and the correspondence theory of truth. These contemporary idealists oppose scientific realism, asserting that we *create* experience, either in the mind, or in analytic conversation, or in both. Depending on the degree of radicalism, these views are a return to the idealism of the 18th-century philosopher Berkeley, for whom the subject was the only source of knowledge. As ontologies, these idealisms imply that the real is the mental; as epistemologies, they claim that we know only our own mental or conversational products, whatever we *make* or create. These views include a coherence theory of truth, according to which truth inheres in a whole system of beliefs. A theory is true if it hangs together, both logically and aesthetically.

Prominent proponents of psychoanalytic idealism include constructivist Hoffman (1983, 1991, 1992a), narrativists Spence (1982) and Schafer (1983), and fictionalist Geha (1993). Hoffman (1991) considers his view a relativist one, and by constructivism he means not only a challenge to the "naive patient" fallacy and the blank screen but a more general epistemological position. He now calls his position "critical constructivism" (Hoffman, 1992b, 1993). "Experience," he explains, "taken as a whole, is partially constituted by what we *make* of it, retrospectively, in the context of interpretation, and prospectively, in the context of experience-shaping actions" (1993, p. 18, emphasis added). This nuanced constructivism, though intended as a radical critique of traditional views, scarcely belongs with the more extreme views.

Another moderate idealism is that of Schafer (1983). While he thinks the analytic process consists largely of creating narratives, he argues that subjectivity itself sets limits on our narratives: "The introspection narrative tells us that far from constructing or creating our lives, we witness them. It thus sets drastic limits on discourse about human activity and responsibility" (p. 225). Spence's (1982) narrative truth is a more extreme position. In his view, we know nothing in the analytic situation except the narrative constructed by patient and analyst.

Most radical of the current critics of psychoanalytic naive realism, Geha (1993) calls his view "fictionalism." I will let him speak for himself:

Psychoanalysis molds the worlds that it interprets. It creates them; it does not find, uncover, or discover them. An analysis in its entirety constitutes a work of *narrative fiction* composed around all the many familiar texts that surface during the analytic process, from dreams to slips of the tongue. Consequently, psychoanalysis emerges as essentially an enterprise of construction, not *re*construction, or at least not reconstruction of something other than the mind's inventions. (pp. 214–215)

A story corresponds to no exteriorities. It is self-referential. It reflects nothing other than, if you will, the cross-reflections of its own integral elements. Every element of a story is determined—as Gestalt psychology once stressed—by the integration that emerges as the recognized story. That is, elements are located, affected, allowed to affect, and conferred with meaning only within the terms of the story. Every bit of the story is imagined. The book is about itself. (p. 225)

That this view finds an audience in such a highly and widely respected journal as *Psychoanalytic Dialogues* attests to the depth of discomfort analysts have come to feel with scientific realism. "Reality" (the analyst's view) and "distortion" (the patient's view) must still be alive and kicking as acceptable psychoanalytic concepts, either in some external world or in our fictional account of the current psychoanalytic scene, to evoke such drastic theoretical measures. The solipsism inherent in extreme subjectivisms and relativisms becomes, as exemplified in Geha's account, an inescapable *folie à deux*, a shared fiction from which there is no escape, perhaps not even into another fiction.

However, many analytic theorists—including the more moderate psychoanalytic idealists Hoffman and Schafer—are using mixed conceptions of experience. While in his seminal paper, "Introspection, Empathy, and Psychoanalysis," Kohut (1959) emphasized the centrality of introspection and empathy as means of accessing psychological phenomena, he also acknowledged that such empathic and introspective observation can use the findings of the sciences:

It may, of course, sometimes be useful for the psychologist to take his clues from biological findings or principles in order to orient his expectations about what he might observe. The final test, however, is psychological observation itself; and it is erroneous to extrapolate the interpretation of a specific mental state from biological principles, especially if they contradict our psychological findings. (p. 223)

Guntrip (1969) later took exactly this position. Thus both Kohut and Guntrip intended to affirm the centrality of the psychological—whatever is knowable by introspection and empathy—without denying that experience is always the experience of something. They recognized that the nonpsychological sciences with their more external perspectives may provide information to guide us as we search into the meaning of complex mental states.

Stolorow and Atwood (1992) also use a mixed conception of experience as both given and made. Ambiguities persist, however. They, for example, use "experience" primarily as a noun. They refer to "structures of experience" and to the "organization of experience," a central idea in their theory of psychoanalytic intersubjectivity. What do they mean by experience? First, it is the *what* that we structure or organize. This sounds like experience as bare, unprocessed givenness, a logical necessity for an empiricist but a psychological impossibility. At the same time, these authors, phenomenologists rather than empiricists, emphatically endorse Kohut's view that introspection and empathy provide the only access to true psychoanalytic data. We can, therefore, infer that they mean subjectively organized experience, not mere representation of external reality. In addition, their intersubjective theory, like self psychology generally, insists on the constitutive role of the emotional environment on the formation of experience. Some might see this as a contradiction in their theory. A more sympathetic reading sees intersubjectivity theory precisely as an attempt to account for both the external, or contextual, and the internal, or subjective, elements in the creation of personal experience. Their view calls for, if not provides, a conception of experience as always partly organized, as more complex than a simple "blooming, buzzing confusion" (James, 1892, p. 29).

Stolorow and Atwood (1992) also reexamine the notion of unconsciousness, thus raising further questions for psychoanalysis about experience. They outline three kinds of unconsciousness. Their "prereflective unconsciousness" refers to structures of experience—or organizing principles—which are not themselves experience but are instead highly general inferences and expectancies distilled from experience. These structures are unconscious insofar as they work outside awareness, like our basic biological systems when intact and healthy. Within this meaning of unconsciousness, "experience" means the past and present content, available to memory or not, that organizing principles organize. Stolorow and Atwood's second type of unconsciousness, "dynamic unconsciousness," like Freud's dynamic unconscious, contains memories of events and bits of self-knowledge and relational knowledge that were once consciously known. This material then became unconscious because it created conflict for the knower. In the view of Stolorow and Atwood, this knowledge was "sequestered" because it jeopardized needed ties to caretakers or threatened the psychological intactness of the potential knower. Here, too, the idea of experience does not require consciousness. Instead, dynamic unconsciousness requires the disavowal, dissociation, or perhaps repression of events or bits of relational knowledge that have already become experience. Prereflective unconsciousness thus creates dynamic unconsciousness. Not that prereflective unconsciousness is a causal agent; instead "maintaining certain prereflective structures or organizations of experience may require the repression or denial of particular contents" (Atwood, personal communication, 1994). Finally, "unvalidated unconsciousness" contains events, emotions, or elements of self experience that did not find receptive acknowledgment and response from caretakers. In my terms, these unvalidated elements have not fully become experience and now are unavailable for conscious experiencing. (A. Miller, 1990, has written similarly about the need for a witness to trauma. See Chapter 9.) Fully conscious experience is articulable memory both for events and for the emotions that organize them into experience.

Another attempt to conceptualize experience comes from the psychoanalysts involved with infant research. Daniel Stern (1985), for example, describes the development of organized relational experience. The caretaker's influence combines with the infant's inborn and developing capacities for subjective relational experience. The infant's process of forming RIGs (representations of interactions generalized) most clearly and fully qualifies for designation as experience. Beebe and Lachmann

(1988), similarly, have contributed a sophisticated model of mutual influence. They imply that experience arises from a combination of outer and inner elements, or what I call the given and the made. This view, and attention to infant studies and early childhood generally, are opposed by proponents of both the empiricist and idealist poles of the continuum. Those who embrace the empiricist (scientific realist) notion of independent or objective fact waiting to be registered are critical of Daniel Stern's work because it focuses on experience as process, as something that develops. Those who lean toward the idealist, or social constructivist, end of the spectrum are critical of infant studies because they rely on assumptions about universality, reality, human nature, or innate capacities, assumptions that sit uncomfortably with the idea that most or all of what we know is singly or jointly a construction, narrative, or fiction.

Ogden's (1989) *The Primitive Edge of Experience* illustrates the need to make our ideas of experience clear and consistent. I find his uses of the term "experience," while often evocative, confusing when taken together. He speaks, for example, of a "schizophrenic fragmentation wherein there is very little of a self capable of creating, shaping, and organizing the internal and external stimuli that ordinarily constitute experience" (p. 196). Here he uses a conception of experience as stimulus, much as scientific empiricists, unequivocal realists, and classical behaviorists do. On the other hand, he speaks throughout of complex experiences like that of ambivalence. He attempts to expand the Kleinian "positions" by speaking of depressive, paranoid–schizoid, and autistic–contiguous forms of organized experience. He eloquently formulates the analytic task:

> As analysts, we attempt to assist the analysand in his efforts at freeing himself from forms of organized experience (his conscious and unconscious "knowledge of himself") that entrap him and prevent him from tolerating the experience of not knowing long enough to create understandings in a different way. The value of developing new ways of knowing lies not simply in the greater self-understanding one might achieve, but as importantly in the possibility that a wider range of thoughts, feelings, and sensations might be brought into being. (p. 1)

Combined with a notion of emotional safety that makes the not-knowing tolerable, Ogden's view of the analytic task would be close to mine. He here uses a complex notion of experience as organized and as reorganizing, but he does not do justice to his own rich understanding of experience by defining it as stimuli.

This brief survey illustrates my contention that contemporary psychoanalysis includes objectivist, idealist, and mixed conceptions of experience. Let us now look to the history of philosophy for some clarifications of these conceptions.

EXPERIENCE IN THE HISTORY OF PHILOSOPHY

Although Aristotle distinguished theoretical from practical knowledge (experience), experience as a concept did not enter philosophical argument until the late Middle Ages with Roger Bacon (d. 1292), who viewed experience as an antidote to authority (Copleston, 1950). Likewise, the philosopher William of Ockham (d. 1349)—best known for "Ockham's razor," or the principle of parsimony—argued that we would never know some realities, like the existence of freedom, by authority or reason alone, but only because experience forced us to recognize them. Thus, without using the 20th-century term, Ockham introduced the notion of "the given," or of the "givenness," of knowing.

Later the Renaissance philosopher and scientist Francis Bacon (d. 1626) distinguished between *mere experience* and *true experience* (Copleston, 1950). Mere experience is like common sense and involves grasping at whatever sense we can make out of what comes our way. True experience, on the contrary, is scientific and planned. It involves turning on the light of theory and making specific tests. Francis Bacon, thus, recognized that the uses of "experience" in ordinary language and daily life often refer to mere givenness, whereas a fuller conception involves the organizing contribution of the knower.

With Descartes, Francis Bacon's conception of two types of experience—"mere" and "true"—fell away. Descartes preached the systematic doubt of all experiential knowledge and the reliance on reason alone, recognizable by its "clear and distinct ideas," as the only reliable criterion. While he acknowledged that the existence of natural phenomena like magnetism could not be inferred from rational systems alone, he insisted that we know such factual matters only when we understand them by reason. We should always hold as suspect "that deceiver," experience.

In reaction, the British empiricists Locke and Hume claimed that all knowledge came through the senses. For them, only what Francis Bacon called "mere experience" deserved our trust. Hume's famous critique of causality—we know only coincidence (what today we call correlation), not cause—relies on this notion of bare, unorganized, reason-free, atomistic experience. Experience became reducible to the perception of the effects of external reality on the immaterial mind.

Ironically, the reduction of experience to sense data evoked an apparently opposing position, Berkeley's idealistic "to be is to be perceived." Sense data are unintelligible; only ideas (today's constructions, narratives, and fictions) are knowable. In this view, experience is the product of intelligence, of creative thought, of the experiencer.

Despite major regressions to Cartesian rationalism, to empiricism, and to empiricist-based idealisms, since the time of Kant, experience has been conceptualized as both given and made. For Kant (1781), the data of sensation and perception become knowledge only as apprehended through the categories, or structures, of the understanding. The mind knows nothing scientific by itself. It is a structured potential for knowing and valuing, or Kant would say, for experience. Like the infant perceptual capacities for relatedness, the categories await the data of perception to form experience, or scientific knowledge. The categories organize the data of perception into experience.

Fascinated with the notion of experience, the American pragmatists may be Kant's truest heirs. Peirce's (1931–1935) work, for example, illustrates the need to give full attention to both the given and the made in experience. On the one hand, he spoke of "brute experience" (vol. 4, par. 172), of "surprise," (vol. 5, par. 51), and of experience as shock (vol. 2, par. 139). This part of experience is change that the subject cannot deny; experience "is the enforced element in the history of our lives" (vol. 5, par. 581). "We experience vicissitudes, especially" (vol. 1, par. 336). Such experience is both source and test of our knowledge.

However, scientific experience was for Peirce, as for Francis Bacon and Kant, much more than "mere" observation:

> Modern students of science have been successful because they have spent their lives not in their libraries and museums but in their laboratories and in the field; and while in the laboratories and in the field they have been not gazing on nature with a vacant eye, that is, in passive perception unassisted by thought, but have been *observing*—that is, perceiving by the aid of analysis—and testing suggestions of theories. (vol. 1, par. 34)

Peirce appreciated both the brute quality of experience and its structured elements. He brought these together in his theory of abduction, according to which science advances when surprising facts impinge on our theories. Then we must be ready to revise our theories, imagine new possibilities, and return to the field and laboratory with new eyes.

For William James experience served as a continual challenge to entrenched theories. Experience, for James, was the *materia prima*, or underlying reality, of everything; things and thoughts, matter and mind, reason and feeling, were just forms of experience (1905). He called this position—which placed him toward the empiricist, or scientific realist, end of the spectrum—radical empiricism. He argued, as had his friend Peirce, that emotion and intuition are part of human life and thus part of human reasonableness. Emotion—or, as psychologists say today, affect—was often for James that part of experience that could or should not be denied. Still, emotion and experience are neither objective (given) nor subjective (made) in themselves. In his words, "subjectivity and objectivity are affairs not of what an experience is aboriginally made of, but of its classification. Classifications depend on our temporary purposes" (p. 74). So, for example, I may treat my suffering as objective: "I have a pain in my foot," or as subjective: "I feel miserable," depending on whether my purpose is to gain doctoring or sympathy. The experience itself, for James, is neither given nor made, it just is. This doctrine of pure experience led to comparisons between James and European phenomenologist Husserl. For emotions, James continued,

> the relatively "pure" condition lasts. In practical life no urgent need has yet arisen for deciding whether to treat them as rigorously mental or as rigorously physical facts. So they remain equivocal; and, as the world goes, their equivocality is one of their conveniences. (p. 76)

James saw experience as the complete substratum, as the blooming, buzzing confusion to be organized by human purposes.

Philosophical hermeneutics has developed a different approach to the problem of experience. In Gadamer's version, it eschews the questions and disputes of traditional epistemology and criticizes its attempt to derive experience from subjectivity. In other words, Gadamer rejects the whole Cartesian enterprise of deriving reality from mind and the empiricist philosophies based on the same dualistic and individualistic assumptions. (The traditional epistemological project in psychoanalysis has recently received a cogent critique from Stolorow and Atwood, 1992, under the rubric of "the myth of the isolated mind.") Any attempt to demarcate the proportions of the given and the made in experience is, for those who thinks hermeneutically, wrongheaded and destined to fail.

Instead, Gadamer replaces Dilthey's empathy—the effort to enter another's experience, to contact another's unities of meaning—with his own view of understanding emergent from conversation. In Gadamer's (1991) words:

> We say that we "conduct" a conversation, but the more genuine a conversation is, the less its conduct lies within the will of either partner. Thus a genuine conversation is never the one that we wanted to conduct. Rather, it is generally more correct to say that we fall into conversation, or even that we become involved in it. The way one word follows another, with the conversation taking its own twists and reaching its own conclusion, may well be conducted in some way, but the partners conversing are far less the leaders of it than the led. No one knows in advance what will "come out" of a conversation. Understanding or its failure is like an event that happens to us. Thus we can say that something was a good conversation or that it was ill fated. All this shows that a conversation has a spirit of its own, and

that the language in which it is conducted bears its own truth within it—i.e. that it allows something to emerge which henceforth exists. (p. 383)

We might ask Gadamer whether he means that understanding can do without a conception of subjective experience. Perhaps the prejudices he considers so valuable in the effort to understand are a kind of organized subjective experiencing. Nevertheless, he raises for psychoanalysis the possibility that understanding is more than empathy, that our focus on experience avoids our historical and intersubjective "embeddedness" (Stolorow & Atwood, 1992). Gadamer prods us to develop a more thoroughly relational conception of experiencing, or to drop the idea of experiencing.

Since, however, experience as a word and a concept is everywhere in psychoanalysis, keeping Gadamer's criticism in mind, I will suggest some ways to think about it. These ideas are not original, but they need to be made explicit and brought into focus. Bringing them together, however, should make it clearer why neither scientific objectivism nor simple social constructivism is an adequate psychoanalytic epistemology.

EXPERIENCE AS INTERPRETATION

I suggest the following ways to think about experiencing:

1. All experience is both given and made. I do not mean that we can just conceive it either way, like the particles and waves of quantum physics, or the ducks and rabbits of Gestalt theory. Both the given and the made are necessary to constitute experience from any perspective. We cannot usually know the exact contribution of each element, nor can we usually distinguish them neatly from one another. Sometimes the given consists of what has previously been organized; it is, in other words, the relatively given. This mixed conception of experience requires our ability to tolerate ambiguity, the lack of which is illustrated by the controversy over false and recovered memory.

2. Givenness refers to brute, at least partly unprocessed,

undeniable events or occurrences. Colloquially we say, "Well, that is a given," that is, the matter is relatively self-evident. Givenness involves the sense that something smacks one in the face like a 40-mile-an-hour wind. Yet the given may include an emotional response or reaction. Givenness may come to include our past organized experiences. The given is a necessary epistemological, logical, and psychological condition for the possibility of experiencing.

3. Making refers to subjective and relational organizing activity, as in the expression, "What do you make of it?" Like Kant's categories of the understanding, but more intersubjectively configured than these, our organizing activity is a second necessary condition for the possibility of any experience. We organize whatever is given in the present emotionally and cognitively from past relational experience. *To experience is to organize the given.* Experiencing is a developing process, not a finished product. Fantasy and dreaming, narrative and construction, are special kinds of organizing activity.

4. Events become experience by emotional processing in an explicit or implicit intersubjective and historical context.

5. To reexperience a feeling or event is to take the past event-transformed-into-experience as the given and to reorganize it, or remake it, according to old or new emotional organizing principles, or modes of emotional inference. We reach, either in inner dialogue or in conversation with another, a new understanding.

6. In psychoanalysis, transference and countertransference (or cotransference) include both the given and the made. Part of the given, for each participant, is the otherness of the other, the brute actuality of a not-me. (Of course, as George Atwood [personal communication, 1994] has pointed out to me, the experience of otherness itself contains elements of the given and the made.) What is "made" is my interpretation or understanding of the other, and of our relation, from my particular vantage point, which includes my emotional history and my theories.

7. The boundary between the given and the made shifts with the intersubjective context. I do not mean that the given and made are poles of experience, but rather that taken together, they comprise experience. A "sense of reality" means that we possess,

at least temporarily, the conviction that the greater portion of our experience lies on the given side (Ferenczi, 1909).

8. As far as bare and unorganized events are either overwhelming or find no responsive emotional context, they may fail to become experience. They remain dissociated, unconscious, and unavailable for integration into a whole experienced life.

9. The distinction between the given and made does not, however, correspond to the continuum between unconsciousness and consciousness. Granted, events and emotions that we find overwhelming or difficult to make sense of—relatively disorganized events—are less likely to come to awareness, but as Freud taught us, they have their ways of surfacing. The given and the made comprise all experience, conscious or unconscious.

To summarize, experience results from the endless and constant interaction, or dialogue, between the given and the made. It emerges within and between the subjectivities involved in any intersubjective field. Individually and together we make sense of (or experience) what is partly brute, unorganized, surprising, or confusing.

Finally, a question that encapsulates this entire problem. Suppose we were to agree to use the word *experience* only as a verb? We could no longer, for example, refer to structures of experience, nor simply to self-experience. We would instead refer each time both to the interpreter's organizing activity and to whatever the interpreter interprets. All experience would become interpretation or organizing activity. I do not believe such a shift in usage will ever catch on, nor can I make this shift consistently myself. Still, the question highlights my central thesis—a thesis widely shared today by all psychoanalysts who acknowledge the influence of the observer on the observed: Whenever we experience, we *do* something—making sense or organizing—*to* something—the given, the partly unorganized, even the chaotic. Psychoanalytic understanding consists of a collaborative effort to make sense of this experiencing.

CHAPTER 7

Affect and Emotional Life

*T*he experience, given and made, that is of interest to a psycho-analytic epistemologist is emotional experience. Human emotional life is what psychoanalysts seek to understand and to heal. If our bodies hurt, we see a physician, at least initially. If our thinking needs improvement, we go to school or read books. If our cars will not run, we take them to a mechanic. If our emotional life feels beyond our power to understand or manage, we may see a psychotherapist. Ordinarily, people take emotional pain as real, and as a reason to seek help. "I don't know why I feel so bad." Yet within psychoanalytic thought emotions have long been seen as less than fully real, as mere epiphenomena, as derivative from those essential motivators, the instinctual drives. Emotions, or affects, were either signals of sexual or aggressive conflicts, or the effects of continuing and unsuccessful unconscious attempts to resolve these conflicts. Since emotion signified trouble, a psycho-analytic cure meant reducing or eliminating emotion. Making the unconscious conscious, full of cognitive insight, should render emotional signals from the unconscious almost unnecessary.

In contrast with this longstanding cognitive emphasis within psychoanalysis, much recent psychoanalytic writing regards affects as psychoanalytic bedrock. Krystal (1988), for example, points to the inability to read and integrate one's own feelings as the core of most psychopathology. Even more recently, Spezzano (1993) has claimed that psychoanalysis, both in Freud and in the work of object relations theorists, has always included a theory of affects. In Spezzano's view, psychoanalysis *is* a theory of affects. Krystal, Spezzano, and other writers provide an important antidote to the cognitive cast of both traditional and some recent psychoanalytic theory. I will consider these contributions in more detail and then suggest some emphases that I believe are crucial to an adequate psychoanalytic theory of emotional life. Last, to illustrate my view of psychoanalytic understanding as making sense together, I will apply my perspectives to an emotion common in human life, envy.

First, however, a word about terminology. "Affect," sometimes "affects" in the plural, is a word psychoanalysts use for primary or fundamental emotions, usually described from an observer's point of view. When emotion belongs to the speaker, that is, when it is subjectively experienced, we call it a feeling. We say "I feel," or "I have a feeling," not "I have such-and-such an affect." Although Krystal (1988) considers "affect" and "emotion" synonymous, the words have different connotations. I prefer to use "emotion" for feelings—to emphasize their character as complex processes rather than as simple entities. Emotions are among Kohut's "complex mental states"—knowable or known only by introspection and empathy. "Affect," on the contrary, lends itself to the atomistic assumptions that I will challenge below. The technical term "affect" adds no meaning to the idea "emotion" and distances us one step further from the feeling or unable-to-feel person. However, when discussing the work of others, I will adopt their language. When advancing my own views, I will use the words "feeling" or "emotion" for subjective emotional experiencing. I will use the words "emotion" or "emotional life" for what we can know only by introspection or empathy, that is, by psychoanalytic methods of observation. "Emotional life" will also refer to the totality or complexity of subjectively experienced feeling, but described as if from outside. In this usage, someone might say, "I don't understand—or I hate—my emotional life."

RECENT PSYCHOANALYTIC WORK ON AFFECT

The important work of Henry Krystal, gathered in *Integration and Self-Healing: Affect, Trauma, and Alexithymia* (1988), provides one entry into recent psychoanalytic thinking on affect. Krystal's contribution includes his view of affect as originally undifferentiated somatic response that, under ordinary conditions, develops by differentiation, articulation, and desomatizing. With adequate parenting, a child learns, during toddlerhood but especially in latency, to bear emotional distress and to know that it will pass. Krystal names the ability to bear the intensity of emotional pain without excessive escapes into anesthetics such as drugs, alcohol, food, or emotional deadness "affect tolerance." He considers bearing affect states and knowing that the future need not resemble the overwhelming past the basic gauge of mental health.

The most common obstacle to acquiring the *ability* to tolerate affect, in Krystal's view, is massive psychic trauma in infancy or adulthood. Working with hundreds of Holocaust survivors taught him—as working with Vietnam War veterans, rape victims, and survivors of severe child abuse was later to teach others—to recognize the freezing, numbing, and blocking, the death-in-life that partly define trauma in adults and in verbal children (Terr, 1990). Courtois (1988), van der Kolk (1984, 1987), Horowitz (1986), and Herman (1992) have described the intrusive symptoms of posttraumatic stress: nightmares, sudden rages, exaggerated startle responses, and flashbacks. Preverbal trauma, on the other hand, as far as we as adults can ever imagine it, is the experience of overwhelming emotion, prolonged into timeless terror, suffered without escape and without help. Krystal believes that the adult residues of such early trauma appear either as emotional frozenness or as panicky responses to any emotion. Emotions are then experienced as the return of the dreaded, timeless, and overwhelming terror of infancy. Krystal, like Spitz and Bowlby before him, sees early loss as the paradigm example of massive infantile trauma. Infants brought to institutions after the war deaths of their mothers struggled in terror, then lapsed into helpless numbness, the precursor of alexithymia.

By "alexithymia," Krystal (1988) means "patients' impaired ability to utilize emotions as signals to themselves" (p. 243). The emotional life of alexithymic patients is usually somatic, unverbalized, undifferentiated, and vague. Such people do not recognize emotion as emotion, in themselves or in others. Instead they may become physically ill, or just numb. Therapy, for these patients, involves recognizing, differentiating, and desomatizing affect. Krystal sees affect itself—even painful emotional states—as constructive and useful.

Given the theoretical and clinical fruitfulness of Krystal's work, my differences may seem minor, but they have extensive theoretical and practical implications. First, extensive infant research, as summarized by Tronick (1989), has found facial responses in newborns that correspond to anger, fear, joy, curiosity, and so on. If emotional responsiveness is originally so varied, then the question becomes, what has happened to that emotional life in people who become alexithymic? Perhaps we must see trauma as shutting down what already exists, rather than as interfering with developmental paths of affect differentiation and desomatization.

The second area in which I differ from Krystal concerns his view of emotion as an internal matter. While he acknowledges both environmental influences on the developed ability to bear affect and the effect of externally perpetrated trauma on emotional life, he considers affect regulation primarily an individual task and mental health a matter of the individual's ability to master this task. Similarly he considers trauma, particularly in infancy, an overwhelming private experience of timeless terror. A shift within Krystal's theory to a relational perspective on human nature, development, health, and pathology would place his work in the center of current psychoanalytic thinking.

In this vein, Stolorow et al. (1987) hold that the intersubjective field shapes and maintains affect. Drawing on Krystal's work, they highlight the extent to which the degree of affect tolerance, for example, depends on the ways the person's parents responded to their child's emotions. More broadly, emotional life takes shape as a person's automatic response to a history of parental response to his or her emotional expressions. In adulthood in general, and in treatment in particular, emotional life, shaped by the person's relational history, similarly develops and heals in mutual interchange.

Stolorow and Atwood (1992) see trauma itself in intersubjective terms. They hold that the shocking and painful affect becomes unbearable and overwhelming because the child finds no understanding and comforting response: "Pain is not pathology. It is the absence of adequate attunement and responsiveness to the child's painful emotional reactions that renders them unendurable and thus a source of traumatic states and psychopathology" (p. 54). For example, a patient who at age 8 had lost a favorite uncle to an airplane crash needed his parents to attend to *his* feelings and worries, not only to their own grief. Analysis provided this patient with the opportunity, an emotional "second chance," to find the attuned responsiveness to his emotional states that could make these states less terrifying and more bearable.

From a relational point of view, Spezzano (1993) has attempted to remedy what he sees as the psychoanalytic neglect of affect since Freud and to integrate a theory of affect into psychoanalysis. His account makes it clear that Freud developed and used a theory of affect.

Similarly, Spezzano shows that the object relations theorists in Britain (especially Fairbairn and Winnicott) and in North America (Loewald, 1980) included a theory of affects in their thinking and that it enriched Freud's theory of affects. At the same time, Spezzano believes that by placing structural theories in the center of their thought, Freud and these theorists obscured and marginalized their psychoanalytic theories of affect. Spezzano's own contribution, as he sees it, is to correct this misunderstanding by making explicit his claim that psychoanalysis *is* a theory of affects. From this point of view he claims that human psychology consists of "shifting dialectical arrangements of affective states" (p. 214) and that the "full development of affect is what psychoanalysis seeks" (p. 215). In Spezzano's view of psychoanalytic cure:

> Within the analytic holding environment, the analysand gets a second chance to achieve competence in using affects as information about his unconscious psychic activity, especially his processing of contacts with others. Repeated experiences of competent affect regulation within the transference give the patient the material with which to construct a self-representation that sustains a sense of perceived affective competence. The conviction that one can competently regulate one's affective life is a state of well-being. (p. 216)

Although he does not mention the work of the intersubjectivity theorists, Spezzano explains that he sees affect as intersubjectively regulated and maintained. He also explains that his theory of affect is not purely cognitive or even representational. Additionally, he captures one form of what I will call "emotional memory" (see Chapter 8):

They [referring to Dreyfus & Wakefield, 1988] portray the process here as more of a representational one than I want to do. I am trying to get at a different situation from the one in which a representation of the father or mother becomes the prevailing object representation and so casts an emotional tone on the child's whole psychological life. . . . A metaphorical way to grasp this notion is imagine that the heat of south Florida could get inside a child who grew up in such a climate and he would always feel oppressively hot. If a child's pain, loneliness, anxiety, or grief is allowed to persist too often and too long, then that affect or blend of affects comes to be the way that child feels all the time. (p. 225)

Despite my admiration for Spezzano's carefully nuanced work, I think it involves, as does the work of Tomkins (1963) and Krystal (1988), an atomistic treatment of single primary affective states, such as excitement, as underlying prime matter (the given). These views suggest the existence of original or fundamental affects, which, like the elements of the periodic table, may combine, but that we can study in isolation. Emotions, in such a view, are like the empiricist's bits of sense data, lacking the complexity and relational meaning that they should have if, as Spezzano holds, they are intersubjectively regulated and maintained. Relational and inter-subjective experience comes later developmentally in these views, and organizes what is given.

These affect theorists (Tomkins, Krystal, and Spezzano), in their yearning for theoretical elegance and simplicity, may also fall into the trap of reductionism. Classical drive theorists insisted that "it all came down to" sexuality and aggression; Greenberg (1991) replaces those drives with effectancy and safety. Similarly, the affect theorists (e.g., Krystal and Spezzano) hope to find a simple principle of explanation for human emotional life. Like Freud, they sometimes imply that the goal of human life is to seek pleasant affect states and avoid unpleasant states. Yet Aristotle explained long ago that pleasure and pain are byproducts of human activity, not ends in themselves. Pleasure and pain are qualities of experience, not things in themselves. The oversimplification involved in reducing emotions to states or things belongs to what Whitehead (1925) called "the fallacy of misplaced concreteness." Ironically, the reverse side of this fallacy is too much abstraction. The affect theorists also fall into this trap. An abstraction called "affect" becomes a general principle of explanation. Such abstraction breaks up emotional complexity, creating the myth of the isolated affect, isolated from context and emotional complexity.

Infant studies (e.g., Daniel Stern, 1985; Tronick, 1989) allow us to see human nature in less reductionistic ways. Possessing extensive relational and organizational capacities, infants are born with differentiated and complex emotional lives. I wonder whether babies may not already have several months of prenatal emotional-relational experience that they continue to reorganize in the face of so much that is new. We might imagine that even before birth, a baby has absorbed from the mother a capacity or incapacity to contain anxiety, for example, or a sense that comforting and calming are or are not possible. From the beginning, the intersubjective situation is the home of emotional life. This field both organizes and gives meaning to emotion.

Perhaps Spezzano thinks that in order for affect (like instinctual drive) to be taken seriously in psychoanalysis, it must precede relatedness developmentally. Unfortunately, although his general perspective is clearly relational, adopting the view that affect precedes relatedness may place Spezzano among those who believe that the sources of motivation are found primarily or exclusively in the patient. Yet a fully relational view of psychoanalysis, one that sees even emotion as constituted in relatedness, does not discount affect. Instead it sees people as continually attempting to make sense of the complex emotional life that they always live in implicit and explicit relatedness to others. My thinking stresses the inherently complex and relational nature of emotional life. With this complexity recognized, I agree with Spezzano that emotional life is psychoanalytic bedrock—the *what* that we seek to understand.

EMOTIONAL LIFE AS COMPLEX AND RELATIONAL

As an antidote to the views discussed above, I wish to emphasize two essential features of emotion: its complexity and its dependence on historical and present contexts of relatedness. First, let us consider the complexity of emotional life.

Emotional life, an irreducibly complex process, requires an epistemology that resists the urge to oversimplify. Relational history makes understanding emotional life an intricate task. We continually organize and reorganize in layers of meaning. Psychoanalysis has long recognized this complexity by referring to multiple function (Waelder, 1936) and overdetermination (Freud, 1910). According to the principle of multiple function, any psychic phenomenon—a dream or a symptom, for example—may serve many psychological purposes at once. Overdetermination, similarly, means that any psychic event has many causes. More recently, Kohut (1977) called psychoanalysis the depth psychological study of "complex mental states" (p. 244). He meant to insist that psychological life, understood in depth, is never simple or reducible to mental atoms.

When we attempt to extract an "affect" from the continuity and complexity of any emotional life, and use that affect to explain something, we make two mistakes. First, we abstract and extract what is inextricable. Second, we may violate the integrity of the person's experience. Although some of this violence is unavoidable, patients often point it out to us. When we attempt to help a patient articulate a feeling, we often hear: "But that's not all," or "It's more than that," or "It keeps changing."

One effect of the psychoanalytic tendency to speak of single emotions has been the focus on ambivalence and its acceptance as a model of mental health. In this view we are always torn between love and hatred, conceived as two basic and simple affects. We must learn to feel both toward the same person at the same time. On the contrary, I see emotional life as originally complex. It makes more sense to wonder how it disintegrated, how it became oversimplified. How did the responses in a given family bring a child to feel that loving a parent was incompatible with anger, or disappointment, or interest in something else besides the parent? How did the child develop the conviction that feeling itself was dangerous to significant ties?

However, isolation or dissociation of some emotions from the whole of emotional life is only one form of difficulty. Many emotions, like shame and dread, are themselves internally layered. Shame involves self-hatred in the face of the explicit or implicit other's perceived or expected disapproval. It is complex, often multiply layered, and usually continuous with moments of more intense pain. People sometimes say, "I'm ashamed that I'm ashamed about this." Likewise the feeling of dread involves both emotional memory and an expectation of further pain or terror, and it usually includes a sense of depressive helplessness.

A second essential feature of emotional life is its relational character. Emotions are responses to relational events or needs, and emotional expression is an attempt to connect, or to regulate connection, with another. The social smile in infants is a *social* smile. Smiling and crying are methods of "object seeking" (Fairbairn, 1952). Any thoroughly relational theory of human nature or psychoanalysis must treat emotional life in that context. Emotional experience begins, continues, and heals in specific intersubjective contexts. When emotional experience is presented as independent of context—psychiatry speaks of "inappropriate affect," for example—this may mislead us into thinking of emotion as mere internal signal. Instead, from the perspective of intersubjectivity theory, we see the emotional expression of the moment as formed by relational history and as evoked or triggered by the intersubjective field of the present. Its reference to the future often consists in the expectation that the relational experience of the future will resemble that of the past, but it includes an anxious hope that someone will respond differently.

Not only complex and relational, emotional life is emotional. This apparent tautology is important only because both psychiatric and psychoanalytic languages have attempted to describe and work with emotion as if it were a cognition or an instinctual derivative. In either case, it is viewed as residing in the individual. On the contrary, I see emotion as a primarily noncognitive and nonverbal relational response. It can be linked to cognitions or schemata, but it has its own reality. Even the language of intersubjectivity theory has been ambiguous on this issue. The talk of "organizing principles" (Stolorow et al., 1987), representation (Beebe & Lachmann, 1988), and schemata (Fosshage, 1994),[*] has a cognitive cast that may deny to emotion a reality of its own and a prominent place in psychoanalytic discourse. Consequently, I speak of "emotional organizing principles" and "emotional modes of inference." Pre-

---

[*]Fosshage (1994) strives for balance by speaking of affective–cognitive schemata.

cisely because these are emotional, they usually operate in such an automatic manner that identifying them is difficult.

The tendency in psychoanalysis toward cognitive formulations becomes even more prominent when we describe our clinical work as making the unconscious conscious, as illuminating unconscious organizing principles, or as clarifying representations or schemata. I think the failure of psychoanalysis to grant emotion a life of its own may account for the persistence of the widely accepted idea that we do not know how psychoanalysis heals. None of the official explanations provides an answer to why it works when it works, and why it does not when it does not. The problem is, as Ferenczi knew well, that psychoanalysis is emotional medicine for emotional ills. Ideas, insights, interpretations, and other cognitive approaches may support emotional healing, but they do not provide it. Recognizing this painful truth, Italian psychoanalysts like DiChiara (in Nissim-Momigliano & Robutti, 1992) suggest that only if the analyst can find room inside herself or himself for *this* patient is there any hope. Similar ideas come from such Ferenczi descendants as Balint, Kohut, and the Ornsteins (cf. Orange, 1995) and from the independent British tradition (i.e., Suttie, Fairbairn, Guntrip, Bowlby, and Winnicott).

Perhaps our leaning toward cognitive expressions comes in part from the painful emotional experience for the analyst that successful analytic treatment requires. We cannot, as Gadamer (1991) reminds us, stand back if we are to understand. We must enter and participate in the emotional life we and our patients create together in the intersubjective field. This draining work requires a depth and intensity of involvement not captured by cartoons of analysts sitting behind patients and taking notes. So we look for words and ritual to drain off some of the emotional intensity and to dilute our connection to our patients. Nevertheless, our patients pay the price for our distancing and for our reluctance or inability to be emotionally available. Such availability means a readiness for a complex and emotional relationship.

If emotional life truly is complex, relational, and "emotional," then certain clinical consequences follow. One is that our patient's "Yes, but . . ." may not be defensive but instead may be a plea for a fuller understanding of "complex mental states" (Kohut, 1959). If we believe that emotion really differs from cognition, then we will distinguish emotion and cognition in talking with patients and support a respect for the contribution of each to a whole human life. We will show regard for a "sense of things"—ours or the patient's—whether or not this sense is verbalizable. In a Winnicottian spirit, we will make more room in many psychoanalytic treatments for art, music, and poetry as means of creating a shared emotional life. We will also have less need to reduce these "forms of feeling" (Hobson, 1985) to any form of cognition or insight.

I will now provide an example of understanding an emotion as a complex, relational–historical, and truly "emotional" matter. The instance of envy as embedded in shame highlights the contrast between reductionism and the psychoanalyst's attempt to discover complex psychological configurations.

ENVY AND SHAME

According to the 1971 edition of the *Oxford English Dictionary*, in the 14th and 15th centuries "envy" meant "malignant or hostile feeling" and "active evil, harm, mischief." In recent centuries, it has come to have the more specific meaning "the feeling of mortification and ill-will occasioned by the contemplation of superior advantages possessed by another." While Freud used the more current meaning, especially in his writings on the psychology of women (Freud, 1925), the strain in psychoanalysis represented by Melanie Klein and Otto Kernberg harkens back to the earlier meanings. In this view, human constitutional aggression and innate destructiveness are manifest in efforts to destroy the "good object" just because it is good. Here I wish briefly to review the positions of Klein and Kernberg and to suggest an alternative way to understand envy within the psychoanalytic theory of intersubjectivity.

Melanie Klein (1975) defined envy as hatred directed toward the good object. She believed that children, out of innate aggressiveness, resent their mother's possession of good things, like milk, for example, because the mother has control over the supply and because they therefore must depend on her for it. Infants want to spoil and destroy this goodness because they cannot have it all for themselves. The Kleinian view places the origin of envy squarely within the individual, and it sees that person as progressively isolated by the envy. Both bad and good objects get destroyed, persecutory anxiety increases, and hope is lost as the good possibilities are eliminated.

In a similar vein, Kernberg (1986) describes the envy his "borderline" patients display toward their analysts as resulting from the fact that these patients, like Klein's infants, fear dependency. To protect themselves against their fears of being in a receptive and dependent position, these patients devalue and attack their analysts. In Kernberg's words, "The greatest fear of these patients is to be dependent on anybody else, because to depend means to hate, envy, and expose themselves to the danger of being exploited, mistreated, and frustrated" (p. 220). Kernberg attributes such inability to receive to the reactivation of "oral rage and envy." Often, he observes, this incapability prevents learning inside and outside the analysis. Patients feel that their envy will destroy the analyst and that they therefore cannot face it or move beyond it.

While the Klein–Kernberg view sees envy as always expressing innate aggressiveness and natural hostility, self psychologists often conceptualize envy as the manifestation of a patient's self-experience as deficient, inadequate, or shameful. Kohut (1971) made explicit the connection between shame and envy:

> The intense reactions of such [shame-filled] people to their setbacks and failures, too, are—with rare exceptions—not due to the activity of the superego. After suffering defeats in the pursuit of their ambitious and exhibitionistic aims, such individuals experience at first searing shame and then often, comparing themselves with a successful rival, intense envy. This state of shame and envy may ultimately be followed by self-destructive impulses. These too, are understood not as attacks of the superego on the ego but as attempts of the suffering ego to do away with the self in order to wipe out the offending, disappointing reality of failure. (p. 181)

Envy, then, expresses longstanding feelings of shame and inadequacy, generated—in an immediate instance—by an experience of failure.

Alice Miller (1986) describes envy as a manifestation of pervasive underlying feelings of inadequacy:

A patient once said she had the feeling that she had always been walking on stilts. Is somebody who always has to walk on stilts not bound to be constantly envious of those who can walk on their own legs, even if they seem to him to be smaller and more "ordinary" than he is himself? And is he not bound to carry dammed-up rage within himself, against those who have made him afraid to walk without stilts? In this way, envy of other things can appear, the result of the defense mechanism of displacement. Basically he is envious of healthy people because they do not have to make a constant effort to earn admiration, and because they do not have to do something in order to impress, one way or the other, but are free to be "average." (p. 330)

In contrast to the constitutional aggression theories, Miller sees envy as reactive, as a product of an emotional climate that has deprived a child of healthy pride and self-esteem.

A view grounded in intersubjectivity theory would take the approaches of Kohut and of Miller one step further and see the envy as arising in response to specific and regular patterns of experience in the emotional environment. Envy might arise originally from the experience of failure—itself an intersubjectively generated experience—to which the caretaker responded with condemnation or scorn, compounding the damage. For example, the parent may have pointed out the child's failures to others and/or may have compared the child to a sibling, relative, or neighbor who learned faster or was better coordinated. The child, in response to feeling unworthy and devalued in the eyes of those whose opinions naturally mattered most, forms a pattern of shame-based envy. Every subsequent occasion when someone else possesses something good becomes another indication of the child's failure and worthlessness. Often this envy becomes coupled with a fundamental conviction of being doomed to failure. Then, of course, many failures result, and the invidious comparisons continue.

This type of shame may begin as early as the first year of life. Daniel Stern (1985) views the infant as forming a rudimentary self in the first year, including what he calls the "subjective self" (p. 124ff.). This self is based on affect attunements and involves the infant's recognition of the other's recognition of the infant's emotional experience. I imagine that continual or traumatic misattunements impair the development of a sense of effectancy.

I further suspect that these misattunements form the early foundation for the child's later sense of worthlessness, with its accompanying envious conviction that others always have (are worth) more.

If we attend closely to the relational contexts in which envy occurs, we may find ourselves questioning the innate aggression theory of envy. A patient in his early 30s, for example, who originally sought treatment for panic attacks, became extremely anxious in social situations in which he had to converse with young couples who already owned homes. His envy of homeowners—especially of those whose parents had provided them with the down payment—was a manifestation of his shame and embarrassment over his original "home." His abusive father had abandoned him as a toddler to the care of his alcoholic mother and schizophrenic grandmother, both of whose screams were often audible to neighbors. The shame also reflected his expectation that others would see him as a loser. This patient spent his first 3 years in treatment attempting to convince me that he—the patient—was a truly terrible person and that something was terribly wrong with him. My inability or refusal to adopt the view of him that he assumed I must have provided a new context in which to organize his experience of himself in the presence of others.

Another patient, an incest-and-torture survivor, continually envies the "normality" of her peers. She envies their happiness, their families, their apparent ease. This envy often arises, however, in a specific intersubjective context: She has confided parts of her story and some of her hopeless feelings to a friend or family member, who responds by telling her to let the past go and get on with her life. First she finds herself withdrawing from the would-be advisor, but then she wonders why she cannot follow all this good advice and envies those who seem able to do so. She then enters a period of intense self-loathing; envy is transformed into shame. In treatment, she expects me to experience a similar impatience with her, and she is constantly on the alert for the tiniest signal that I may find her impossible or disgusting.

In a third example, an actress becomes depressed when her peers get roles for which she has auditioned or when they become "household names." She envies their success, their money, their friends, their self-confidence. When she is working as an actress, she experiences little envy and is pleased for others who succeed. Her sense of success, however, never outlasts the current performing engagement. In her family, her performing was never welcome, and, after 15 years and some successes in "the business," her father still asks when she is going to grow up and get a job. Her mother assumes that the patient will create a disaster out of anything she attempts. The envy arises as an expression of shame over her family's and her own expectations of failure. "What's wrong with me?" the patient sobs, assuming I too will believe this is the right question. Her past accomplishments usually seem completely unreal to her.

In treatment, envy of the therapist/analyst may be an expression of this shame. The analyst's education, office, fees, vacations, and even manner of dress may evoke envy linked to the patient's sense of being a hopeless failure. Recently a young man said he envied me my sense of security. Patients often believe their therapists have more knowledge or possessions, better family relationships, and better mental health than they do. While these beliefs often manifest patients' generalized convictions, they also result from our professional demeanor or reserved behavior. The shame-based envy often arises in specific situations of misunderstanding or misattunement. Sometimes I miss the despair in a patient's account of failed attempts to form friendships and intimate relationships. Then the patient may conclude that such matters are easy for me, that I have all these things in abundance, and that I could not possibly understand such a shameful and hopeless case. Close attention to the intersubjective contexts in which envy of the therapist occurs may yield evidence to challenge the innate-aggression theory of envy. The disruptions may evoke generalized emotional organizing principles based in early experiences of self-with-other.

To summarize, I think that it is reasonable to understand envy in most instances as a relational expression of shame, that is, of a severe devaluing of the self. Sometimes it may involve deficits in the sense of self as continuous, times when there is a lapse in a person's ability to retain a sense of the reality of past successes. Envy usually arises when a person compares him- or herself with others to the detriment of the self. It is often specifically triggered by misattunements experienced as meaning that something is wrong with the person. When we as therapists respond to envy in a patient, not as though it were evidence of hatred and aggression, but rather as an expression of the presence within the patient of a sense of self-as-deficient (perhaps in the context of an intersubjective misattunement) the patient will usually feel understood, that her or his self-experience has been treated with respect.

Envy thus serves as an example of my contention that emotional life is inherently complex and relational. The emotion itself is complex, though its intensity can mislead us into seeing it as a simple entity. In addition it has complex ties to a person's whole organization of emotional experience and to the particular relational situation in which it arises. The healing of an emotional life full of envy involves not so much affect tolerance (Krystal, 1988), as it requires that patient and analyst understand together the complex involvement of the patient's basic *emotional* sense of a deficient relational self. When this sense of self becomes stronger and more positive, envy recedes or disappears, and with it much shame.

To sum up, I have argued for replacing an atomistic conception of affects—a too-easy substitute for instinctual drives as the explanatory foundation in psychoanalysis—with an attentiveness to the totality and complexity of a person's emotional life. The details and the history of the particulars are important but only as far as they conduce toward understanding a person's organized emotional "sense of things." We must neither reduce the whole emotional life to the sum of its parts nor mistake the affective trees for the emotional forest.

CHAPTER 8

Emotional Memory

I would unlearn the lingo of exasperation. . . .
I would believe my pain, and the eye quiet on
the growing rose.
                    —THEODORE ROETHKE, "The Longing"

Psychoanalytic understanding requires memory. To make sense of ourselves we need to remember how we came to feel and act as we do. An important problem in contemporary epistemology, however, has been its ahistorical character. The recent psychoanalytic emphasis on the here-and-now and on the collaborative construction of narratives can similarly neglect development and history. Yet a conception of psychoanalytic understanding based in intersubjectivity theory—which views all emotional life as configured by past relational experience, requires an enriched appreciation of remembering.

"Emotional memory," one type of remembering, is any felt residue of the relational past. A situation, a thing, or an event—a separation, a sofa, a graduation—produces emotion in us—fear, anticipation, sorrow—we may not understand. Emotional memory, which names a cluster of ways of knowing, reexperiencing, and expecting, largely noncognitive and nonverbal, has long been known to psychoanalysis. It includes transference, dreams, body memory, vague and particular dreads, many moods, overreactions, and the experiences underlying some forms of repetition. Although the content of emotional memory may be verbal experience, we usually carry such memory in nonverbal forms. Beginning with Freud, psychoanalysts have known that nonverbal experience can carry meaning. The concept of emotional memory provides a way to think about the connections among the phenomena of preverbal and wordless memory. What the phenomena have in common is the continuing emotional effects—conscious or unconscious—of our relational history.

Emotional memory is not necessarily pathological or pathogenic; it is human. We carry our history within us, only a small part of which is cognitively processed. Most experiencing is visceral, emotional, and only partly organized. Relational circumstances— including, of course, the implicitly relational experience of being alone—that somehow resemble earlier ones can trigger or evoke such emotional memory. Close attention to emotional memory, and to those events that evoke it, can expand and deepen our psychoanalytic understanding. It is often emotional memory, not immediately recognizable as memory, that we attempt to make sense of together in analysis.

SOURCES OF THE CONCEPTION
OF EMOTIONAL MEMORY

The notion of emotional memory has obvious antecedents. Several recent philosophers, in contrast to the midcentury reduction of philosophy to linguistic analysis, have insisted that experience includes more than words can express. French philosopher Henri Bergson (1910), for example, emphasized the temporal continuity of experience, as contrasted with the atomist discontinuities so beloved by empiricists. In his words:

> We instinctively tend to solidify our impressions in order to express them in language. Hence we confuse the feeling itself [of temporal duration, for example] which is a perpetual state of becoming, with its permanent external object [the clock], and expressly with the word which expresses this object [time]. (p. 130)

Similarly, Alfred North Whitehead (1948) pointed out the necessary incompleteness of linguistic cognition: "There is not a sentence which adequately states its own meaning. There is always a background of presupposition which defies analysis by reason of its infinitude" (p. 73). Whitehead suggested both humble and proud views of linguistic expression. Language captures only a small part of experience, but language invests the present with the past and renders the past "articulated memory."

Philosopher Michael Polanyi (1958) wrote extensively about *tacit knowledge,* the "more than we can say" that we know. Polanyi spoke of the personal participation of the knower, including what Polanyi called the inarticulate or the "ineffable." Not intending the mystical connotation of the term "ineffable", he used it instead to mean "something that I know and can describe even less precisely than usual, or even only very vaguely" (p. 88). As examples, he cites knowing how to ride a bicycle or how to recognize one's own raincoat. There is no reason, he claimed, for this kind of knowledge to be articulable. The problem, he thought, lies in the common assumption that only what language can articulate counts as knowledge. He cites Wittgenstein's (1921) famous aphorism, "What we cannot speak about [as a verifiable proposition of natural science] we must pass over in silence" (p. 74). This ex-presses, in Polanyi's view,* both the Cartesian devotion to clear and distinct ideas and the modern philosophical allegiance to linguistic clarity. Such clarity comes at a price: The richness of tacit knowl-edge, and its personal character, are lost. In psychology and the other social sciences, Polanyi thought, this becomes an important loss. Not surprisingly, he criticized Freud for his advocacy of scientific detachment in psychoanalysis.

Tacit or inarticulate knowledge includes topographical knowl-edge—the knowing-one's-way-around of a surgeon or a taxi driver—and instrumental knowledge—skills such as diagnostics to be taught and learned by example. Another form of inarticulate knowledge is "our own capacity to distinguish what we know from what we may be saying about it" (p. 91). The "what we know" is existential meaning, an understood but not articulated meaning.

In addition, words themselves have subsidiary inarticulate meaning that includes memory:

> Words convey nothing except by a previously acquired meaning. . . .
> When I receive information by reading a letter and when I ponder

---

*I think Polanyi misunderstood Wittgenstein here. Wittgenstein's *Tractatus Logico-Philoso-phicus* (1921) emphasizes a distinction between saying and showing. Many important realities can be shown.

the message of the letter, I am subsidiarily aware not only of its text, but also of all the past occasions by which I have come to understand the words of the text, and the whole range of this subsidiary awareness is presented focally in terms of the message. (Polanyi, 1958, p. 92)

Polanyi did not directly address the question of emotional knowledge. Still, his notion of "tacit knowledge," knowledge by personal participation in the known, is an important conceptual foundation for what I am calling emotional memory. Not every instance of tacit knowledge is emotional memory. Nevertheless, many bits and pieces of procedural knowledge—the topographical and instrumental skills mentioned above—involve a wordless sense of the relational context in which they were learned. A child learns to tie his or her shoes, to tell time, or to ride a bicycle, for example, in a particular emotional environment, which may be intimate or distant, supportive or scornful. The accompanying emotional memories may become articulable, but most frequently they just continue to form the underlying emotional tone of much adult experience. Perhaps whenever the adult needs to learn something new, he immediately feels "like a klutz" or "like a loser." Another adult may feel awkward or embarrassed every time someone is watching while she ties her shoes. In this example, the tacit knowledge of how to tie one's shoes also includes the tacit knowledge—the intersubjectively formed organizing principle—that one is a failure.

Similarly, Gadamer's philosophical hermeneutics points out the ways in which words only partly express what is unsaid. In a conversation, both speakers and listeners bring a web of preconception—Gadamer's "prejudice"—and tradition, thereby creating a new tradition from their exchange. History and memory thus become the unarticulated bases of all attempts at understanding. In Gadamer's (1991) view, prejudice—preconceived bias—forms the possibility of our knowing anything, especially something new. Memory, tacit or articulate, unconscious or conscious, makes new experience and knowledge possible. Just as we cannot read without prior knowledge of language, we cannot experience our emotional life in the present without the web of felt meaning that we carry from our past.

In "Remembering, Repeating and Working Through," Freud (1914) introduced the idea of repetition as remembering to psychoanalytic thought. He believed that patients usefully enact what they cannot remember directly. They repeat the experiences underlying their symptoms, inhibitions, "unserviceable attitudes," and "pathological character traits" (p. 151). Thus, without having to recognize the sources of their difficulties, patients bring their troubles into the treatment. In Freud's words, "one cannot overcome an enemy who is absent or not within range" (p. 152). The conception of emotional memory, therefore, has its roots deep in the beginnings of psychoanalysis.

Emotional memory, however, differs from, and includes more than, repetition. The notion of repetition—usually referring to repeated patterns of behavior or interaction—describes people from an external viewpoint. *The idea of emotional memory,* on the contrary, *highlights the subject's experience,* felt now as if it were then. In analysis we commonly find that the intersubjective field both evokes and develops such remembering. Recently I told a patient that I had visited and liked her hometown. In response, she began to tell stories of having been tormented and terrorized by older girls in junior high school. She commented that she had not remembered these experiences for many years. We could link her terror then to the rage she now feels at some kinds of mistreatment. Perhaps it was my venturing even a mild feeling about her hometown that opened up her access to emotional memory.

Ferenczi, too, alerted us to the physical–emotional ways that we carry our history. His work with survivors of incest (Ferenczi, 1933) significantly anticipated what today's clinicians (e.g., Horowitz, 1986; Herman, 1992) understand about post-traumatic stress. He recognized that experiences of confusion and shame could live on in a person's experience. For instance, Ferenczi (1929) found that a hated child could encode this early relational experience into a lifelong desire to die or a reduced desire to live. He noted that such emotionally encoded convictions were impervious to talk therapy alone, and he wondered what else might help.

Ferenczi (1932) thought that adults have two systems of memory: subjective memory (emotional and bodily) and objective memory (of external events). Infants, on the contrary, have only subjective and bodily sensations and responses, and thus only subjective memory. He believed that this subjective memory continues to predominate for the first 3 or 4 years of life. Yet at moments of trauma, people of all ages register experience in this mode. "The 'memory' remains fixed in the body and only there can it be awakened" (pp. 260–261). Ferenczi thought it unreasonable to expect that people would directly and consciously remember such early experience or trauma. Instead, they reexperience or subjectively remember it in analysis, and in this way traumatic memory becomes accessible. Ferenczi's work identifies the theoretical implications of (1) taking trauma seriously and (2) describing developmental differences in ways of experiencing and knowing.

Much later, Hans Loewald (1960b) described memory as inherently relational, "inextricably interwoven with experiences of separation, loss, object withdrawal, or cessation of satisfying external interactions" (p. 160). He distinguished between representational and enactive remembering, explicitly including more than acting out and transference repetitions in enactive remembering. He held that enactive remembering is characteristically unconscious:

> From the point of view of representational memory, which is our ordinary yardstick, we would say that the patient, instead of *having* a past, *is* his past; he does not distinguish himself as rememberer from the content of his memory. (p. 165)

Loewald noted that increased affect interferes with representational memory because the distance required for representation is usually absent. He also thought that moods are a form of nonrepresentational remembering, citing anniversary reactions as an example.

Similarly, Bollas (1987), of the British Independent School speaks of "existential memory" and of the "unthought known." He considers moods, the search for transformational experience, and the handling of the self as forms of memory. Moods, he believes, create a "conservative object." This object "preserves a self state that prevailed in the child's life just at the moment when the child felt he lost contact with the parents" (p. 113). Bollas thinks that as adults we seek transformational experience that changes self-experience by altering our physical and emotional environment in the same way that caretaking, the "transformational object," did for us as infants. Even our treatment and handling of ourselves as adults is a way of remembering the ways—gentle or harsh, for example—caretakers managed us as children.

By "existential memory" Bollas means "nonrepresentational recollection," memory registered in one's being. In his words, "a person's character is a subjective recollection of the person's past, registered through the person's way of being with himself and others" (1987, p. 35). More recently, Bollas (1989) has characterized what he calls "ego structure" as memory. He claims that "infants do internalize the mother's actual idiom of care, which is a complex network of 'rules for being and relating' " (p. 195). The child, he believes, organizes these relational rules and assumptions into a deep personal structure. He continues:

> Isn't ego structure a form of memory, and its structure a testimony to the logic of its formation rather like a building recollects an architect's intent? If so, this type of memory is operational and structural and not representational and recollective. (p. 195)

My thinking about emotional memory, though not tied to object relations theories, is heavily indebted to the writings of Bollas. His implicit rejection of mind–body dualism provides a basis for beginning to examine the memorial character of all human experience. His expression "somatic knowledge" (1987, p. 282) conveys an appreciation for the way experience encodes itself in our whole being as memory. He thus expresses anew the relational theorists' conviction that relational experience becomes self experience. In general Bollas expresses recognition and respect for "that part of the psyche that lives in the wordless world" (1987, p. 3).

Likewise, Joyce McDougall's (1989) thinking points toward that presymbolic and largely nonrepresentational knowledge that I am calling emotional memory. She studies the memorial quality of psychosomatic illness, the ways we carry our past in our bodies. Emotion, she claims, *"is essentially psychosomatic"* (p. 95). She has dropped the term "alexithymia" (Krystal, 1988) because of its exclusive concentration on the missing ability to verbalize emotion, and she examines instead the positive content of body memory. Here is an eloquent example of her thinking:

> The extreme fragility, observable in the course of analysis, of the narcissistic economy of many addicted, disaffected, and somatizing analysands, linked to the incapacity to contain and to elaborate verbally numerous affective experiences, provides hypothetical answers regarding possible etiological factors. At the level of recall, there is frequently reference to a family discourse that promulgated an ideal of inaffectivity, as well as a condemnation of imaginative experience. Beyond these elements of conscious recall I have sometimes been able to reconstruct with my patients the existence of a paradoxical mother-child relationship in which the mother was felt to be out of touch with her child's emotional needs. Perhaps in response to her unconscious fear of her own affective life, she (in the analysand's memory) controlled to the utmost her child's thoughts, feelings, and spontaneous gestures. While we may never know just what transpired in the intimate bodily and psychological exchanges between mother and infant to render emotional experience unacceptable or lifeless, we are able to observe what happens when experiences charged with affect arise in the psychoanalytic relationship. Pulverized affect will sometimes come to light as part of the discovery of a lost continent in the inner psychic world. (pp. 103–104)

McDougall's work illustrates the clinical inquiry and inference needed to use emotional memory in the psychoanalytic situation. She is more inclined than I am to view body memory as pathological and as resulting from a failure of verbalization. In addition, although she speaks the language of drive and discharge, her ideas fit more comfortably in a relational framework. Her work illuminates the effects of intersubjective experience on bodily memory.

Kohutian self psychology has, since its beginnings, attended to knowledge, memory, and experience that extend beyond the realm of language. Kohut (1978b) said that long before he articulated his self psychology, he was "fascinated by the problem of understanding contentless traumatic states" (p. 932). This interest, he said, stimulated his attempts to articulate psychological understandings of music. In his work on music, Kohut distinguished the *content* of a parental communication, accessible to verbalization and secondary processing, from its *form* or the tone. This tone may be "piercing or cutting, heatedly angry, or coldly killing by mortifying distance" (1957, p. 241). Later, Kohut's central conception of selfobject experience conveyed his continued attention to the *wordless connections between humans and their emotional caretakers.* For example, Kohut's identification and articulation of the constitutive developmental function of idealizing—which by its very nature is a wordless and remembered yearning—could only have come from attunement to nonverbal connections and communications.

Finally, the theory of intersubjectivity developed by Stolorow et al. (1987) provides a theoretical framework for emotional memory. Understanding all psychic phenomena as resulting from the interplay of differently organized subjectivities, memory can only be seen as relational. In addition, with Daphne Stolorow (D. Stolorow & R. Stolorow, 1987), these authors suggest that affect forms the core of selfhood, a view that challenges the centrality of representational knowing. The "organizing principles" for which these authors search in their "sustained empathic inquiry" must then be more emotional than strictly cognitive. More recently, Stolorow and Atwood (1992) have reexamined and enriched the psychoanalytic idea of unconsciousness, expanding it to include a conceptual place for parts of one's history that because they were never validated, never became conscious experience. Their theory thus acknowledges the many ways in which early intersubjective experience becomes encoded.

THE CONCEPTION OF EMOTIONAL MEMORY

Emotional memory includes any form or part of experience that largely bypasses cognitive processes and carries significant residues from the intersubjective worlds of the past. Emotional memory has an unmediated quality that makes it feel compelling. Examples include transference, dreams, and attractions to people who resemble our parents. In addition, the study of posttraumatic stress has drawn attention to nightmares, flashbacks, exaggerated startle responses, and rages. Recent awareness of the sequelae of child abuse has also highlighted sexual phobias, impaired body sense, and extreme self-hatred as forms of emotional memory.

Unlike unconsciousness, which is defined by what remains outside awareness, emotional memory concerns what and how a person *does* know. It needs no theory of repression, but requires instead an understanding of the many ways people of any age register and encode their experience (Schachtel, 1959; G. Klein, 1966). The idea of emotional memory does not, however, replace that of unconsciousness; for example, we can have greater or lesser cognitive awareness about a given form of body memory. What a conception of emotional memory can do is explain why making the unconscious conscious has such limited therapeutic efficacy. The emotional memory remains embedded in the person's organizing principles, retaining much of its power until sufficient new relational experience is in place. This new experience in turn becomes emotional memory, which like all emotional memory is only partly articulable.

Developmental psychologists have attempted to describe the emergence of memory. Distinguishing between recognition and recall, these researchers have found that infants can recognize their mother's face in the earliest days and months of life. Babies and toddlers later develop more sophisticated memory capacities (Piaget, 1968). Despite the awareness by Piaget and his followers of sensorimotor memory, they primarily studied the development of cognitive memory, both recall (for Piaget, evocation) and recognition. Sensorimotor memory, which is so strongly related to what I am calling emotional memory, became for the Piagetians primarily a precursor of the fully representational memory of symbolically organized schemata (cf. Jones, 1995).

More recently, in the large literature on infant cognitive and relational capacities, Daniel Stern (1985) has provided a less cognitive cast to the study of early memory with his RIGs (representations of interactions generalized). Stern (1988) distinguishes between specific and prototypic memories, seeing the latter as representations that endure:

> Since the representation is an abstracted accumulation—undergoing constant updating—of historical events, it will be a very conservative force upon interpreting any currently lived-event (the interpersonal

reality). In other words, past experience will have enormous weight in the construction of present subjective experience. People will repeat the same behaviors, selective inattentions, interpretation, etc. This is, in fact, the single stickiest problem in therapy. (p. 51)

This conservative function of memory resembles the view of memory presented by Piaget and Inhelder (1973), who believed that memory in the wider sense (our total and organized store of knowledge) has a significant influence on the particular memories we retrieve (memory in the strict sense). In the words of Flavell (1977), "what the head knows has an enormous effect on what the head learns and remembers" (p. 189). We may carry these proto-typic memories all the time, as Daniel Stern believes, or they may arise only in response to triggers or stimuli. According to Stern, these representations, or prototypic memories—in contrast to the verbalizable content-laden specific memories (Piaget's memory in the strict sense)—carry "the full weight of past history" (p. 51). Perhaps emotional memory consists in part of these RIGs (repre-sentations of interactions generalized), but often in a less cognitive, less organized, and more directly sensorimotor way than Stern's account suggests. Stern (1983) has acknowledged, however, that affect memory is "only roughly translatable into a language code" (p. 17). I think Stern's view is consistent with the depth of convic-tion with which adults hold emotional and relational organizing principles. Stern's work also explains why the experience behind these principles can be difficult, if not impossible, to articulate.

Emde (1983), another infant researcher, writes of a "pre-representational" affective core of the self. It "guarantees our continuity of experience across development in spite of the many ways we change" (p. 165). Emde finds several sources of evidence for an affective core of the self. A common-sense argument is our belief that we know another to the extent that we contact the other's emotional life. In addition, he mentions research showing that similar dimensions of quality (pleasure/unpleasure) and quantity (intensity) characterize emotional life in infants, chil-dren, and adults. He further points out that cross-cultural studies and infant research have found similar manifestations of emo-tional life. Emde concludes that because affects are similar throughout life and across cultures and research modalities, they represent a core experience. He also notes the evocative effect of the mother's emotional availability. He takes the tendency of infants toward "social referencing"—the infant or toddler checks the mother for emotional responses in situations of uncertainty—as evidence for a predominant affective core of the self. If Emde is correct, emotional memory would consist largely of prerepresentational encoding of relational experience. Neither Emde nor I believes, however, that such sensorimotor and affective encoding stops with the acquisition of language. Instead, I think, *such tacit memory continues to be the core of our knowing, not the precursor of representational, or symbolic, cognition.* I thus prefer Polanyi's "inarticulate knowledge" or my "emotional memory" to Emde's *pre*representational self, but I value Emde's emphasis on such knowledge as the core of selfhood.

In summary, the study of emotional memory, both in theory and in clinical practice, teaches a new respect for knowing that precedes, underlies, and extends beyond the verbal realm. It teaches us to presume that all experience has meaning and history, even—or especially—when it cannot be adequately articulated. For clinicians, this means we must often be content with partial understandings. We bring to our work and to our patients' search for self-knowledge the attitudes of understanding parents, who know that their child's experience somehow makes sense but that good-enough understanding is often the best possible. This fallibilistic attitude works well if the tie to the analyst is strong and if a safe place has been created for the patient's emotional life in the analysis. In turn, the analyst's emotional receptivity to and respect for both verbal and nonverbal aspects of the patient's experience can strengthen the therapeutic bond.

CLINICAL EXAMPLES OF EMOTIONAL MEMORY

Terry came to treatment in her early 20s having heard her psychology professor speak of the successful treatment of incest survivors. She was born in South America, where she lived until she was 7 years old. Her mother's family practiced revengeful sorcery extensively. At the age of 4, Terry was left in their care when both of her parents moved to the United States to find work. When she and her older sister joined their parents 3 years later, their violent and alcoholic father frequently beat her mother and sister, and he raped Terry. Terry could say this much about her history when she began treatment. A few months later she dropped out of school, feeling that everyone could see that she was actually an animal and not human. Occasionally, when she could not reach me, she would write what she was feeling. Here is an example:

> *My poor little cells are screaming for freedom again. My whole body is shaky. I woke up with a physical and emotional pain in my gut. I feel that same terrible, devastating feeling of loss. As though the most vital part of me is dead; so why get up? To tell you the truth I'm pissed at myself for having gotten up, because it means I'm going to live through today. And for what?! There are tears in my eyes and pain in my soul. I do feel as though something very precious had died or is lost. I don't feel real or whole. The only real thing I feel is this overwhelming sadness and pain. . . . I look so fucking normal on the outside. Meanwhile in the inside there's a volcano, because what I see is darkness, dirtiness, ugliness. I see a type of torture chamber, with pieces of myself on several different torturing gadgets; stretching, turning, pulling. With ugly, threatening faces sneering at my fragments and laughing at their futile attempts to escape. . . . I look out from a small crack on the dungeon's wall and see people singing, playing, laughing. And I yearn so much to be one of them.*

Terry sometimes found notes in her handwriting from classes she could not recall having attended. She reported that friends and family told her she was like different people. Sometimes she was adult and competent, sometimes curled up in a fetal position in a corner, sometimes flirtatious, sometimes sobbing for days at a time, sometimes enraged and violent, though usually only toward herself. Often she has desperately wanted to take a large knife, cut open her middle, and get something terrible and disgusting out.

Terry has read *Sybil* and knows that she resembles people diagnosed as having multiple personalities. Over her 5 years in treatment, what has helped most, however, has been encouraging her to construe her diverse feelings and states as emotional memory. This process has not made everything verbalizable, but it has had several other effects. She has gained access to more of her horrifying history. She has come to understand that there are reasons for her feelings and responses that she formerly had characterized as crazy. As a result, she is now less inclined to blame herself, and she is less suicidal. Any sense of being loved, however, is dangerous for her. Terry had loved, and felt loved by, her abusive father. When she and her boyfriend decided to get married, she "freaked out" and expected him to hurt her. Once she understood this as remembering, she calmed down remarkably.

Because Terry had suffered severe trauma at the hands of both women and men, a complicated transference emerged. She experiences me as both benevolent and as highly dangerous. Perhaps the emotional bond appears to promise safety, thereby evoking the memory of other caretakers from whom she might have expected protection. On the other hand, her parents had left her in the care of women who mistreated her severely. Her memories of these horrors surface in her terror of me, a physical–emotional terror that a part of her recognizes as unrelated to the actual me. She recoils in fright if I make any unexpected movement. Each year in the spring she disappears from treatment for a month or two. Only recently have we come to understand that spring reminds her of the weather in her South American country, which triggers feelings that I may hurt her and that I will be unable to protect or help her. On the other hand, she feels I am the only person who has always treated her respectfully, who has believed in her worth when she could not.

Terry exemplifies the wordless "unthought known" (Bollas, 1987) of emotional reaction and expectancy. My work with Terry has involved our coming to understand together that some experiences are horrors beyond words.

Some briefer illustrations may further clarify my understanding of emotional memory. A patient who feels immobilized and cannot understand why he is unable to get himself to do anything to improve his life, especially in terms of relationships, came to see this state as memory. His psychotically depressed mother had stayed and raged at his alcoholic and gambling-addicted father. This patient's paralysis preserved both the inability of his mother to change her situation and his attachment to his more affectionate father who loved to sit and watch baseball on television.

Another patient, learning to play bridge, found herself feeling depressed, hopeless, and tearful. Every rational thought went out of her head when her teacher, an older man, criticized her play of the hand or her bidding. She came to recognize that this man's sarcastic and condescending tone closely resembles her father's. She recalled that card-playing in her family had often occasioned these feelings in a similar relational context. Understanding such "overreaction" as emotional memory, she could go ahead and learn to play bridge from someone else. She did not have to understand her feelings as meaning she was now incapable of learning anything or doing anything right.

Another patient, a late adolescent whose principal symptoms are both vague and particular fears and dreads, originally thought she was simply "crazy." Her treatment has often consisted of exploring these fears and dreads as emotional memory. Some of these feelings have antecedents that she can remember cognitively but about which she had never told anyone. We understand her silence as due in part to shame over having been repeatedly molested as a child. In addition, she had never seen a connection between what happened then and what she is feeling now. Her emotional memories encode in particular the relational experience of having no one to rely on and of being taken repeatedly to the home of the abuser even after she had told a parent about the molestation. She has found that treatment helps because "now I know there are reasons for my feelings even when I can't say them." Also someone knows and cares about what she is feeling, even if no one can change the facts of her history.

IMPLICATIONS

A clinical focus on emotional memory has several advantages. First among these is a positive regard for the patient's experience. Traditionally psychoanalysis has emphasized the negative: the unconscious, the out-of-control, the acting out, the resistance. Now we can attend to what the patient *does* know and begin to explore the many forms of this knowledge. A frequent side-effect of this respect is a gradual reduction in the patient's shame about feelings and needs. One man said that the most helpful intervention in his treatment was my response that it was all right to feel disappointed and that we could learn something from that. Even the shame itself can express a memory. Another patient was so shame-ridden that she would stand up and face the corner of the room when she had to cry. We understand this as remembering her sense of how she had felt as a child when her parents had responded dismissively to her feelings.

Understanding emotional memory also helps explain why symptoms rarely disappear completely and can return under stress. *Our history resides in our whole being.* Insight—even emotional understanding—may mitigate the effects of history, slowly making them manageable and tolerable, but the emotional history remains. What can be healing is the relational experience of safe attachment and of a mutually pursued search for understanding. Such experience creates new emotional memories, new tradition (Daniel Stern, 1991), and new possibilities. Still, no analysis completely removes the effects of rape or child abuse, or keeps the war veteran from terror at the sound of firecrackers. We need not feel that psychoanalysis fails because insight does not remove emotional memory. We cannot expect that it should.

The study of emotional memory may also enhance our understanding of transitional phenomena (Winnicott, 1958). We can see them as expressions of nonrepresentational relational memory. Winnicott thought that the ability to use transitional phenomena showed some history of attachment and was therefore a positive prognostic sign. Similarly, we might see the capacity for transitional experience as one kind of emotional memory and regard its emergence as a sign of progress in treatment. Respect for nonrepresentational modes of knowing and remembering can attune us to such signs of growth.

Attending to emotional memory has other implications for psychoanalytic understanding. Informally we might say that our attention needs to shift, at least in part, from the words to the tune. Many theorists acknowledge that nonverbal elements enter the treatment process and require analysis. Often, however, this is expressed as a concession, betraying again the psychoanalytic bias in favor of verbalization. I believe, on the contrary, that while words can be rich resources for the expression and empathic understanding of emotional experience, and can help patients respect and appreciate their emotional lives, affective memory can be only partly articulated. I also think that the psychoanalytic emphasis on verbalization reflects a Cartesian mind–body dualism. It perpetuates a devotion to the "myth of the isolated mind" (Stolorow & Atwood, 1992) or to Ryle's "ghost in the machine" (1949), conceptualizations that need to be rejected. This renunciation will lead us to avoid characterizing nonverbal expressions of history and development in pejorative terms like "enactment" or "acting out." We can then begin to value and explore the nonverbal expressions and responses of both patient and analyst.

An advantage of emotional memory as a theoretical–clinical conception is its inclusiveness. It regards as resources for psychoanalytic understanding such indicators as tone of voice, startle responses, and facial expression. Many clinical puzzles, about both patient and analyst responses, yield to recognition of the emotional memory involved. According to Peter Lessem (personal communication, 1993), the idea of emotional memory can frequently be a clue in couples therapy to the sources of conflicts and misunderstandings. It can open the way to empathic understanding within the couple and in the therapist. The entry of dissimilar sets of emotional memories into the intersubjective field of the marriage, and into the treatment, is what all concerned need to understand. Emotional memory, in other words, is a significant component, only partly organized and only partly articulable, of the organization of experience.

A correlative concept to emotional memory is "emotional amnesia," a common clinical phenomenon. This occurs in people who have clear, even detailed, recall for past events but no feelings about them. I sometimes work with rape or incest survivors who retain clear memories of what happened, but they cannot feel anything about it. In two instances, these patients have been intensely suicidal. The restoration of emotional memory in such instances becomes the central work of treatment.

Finally, analysts, no matter how well analyzed, are full of emotional memory. Our relational experience, too, has been encoded as the "unthought known" (Bollas, 1987), and it surfaces with every patient in one way or another. This is the "cotransference," that mixture of organizing principles and personal history that always shapes the analyst's experience of the analytic relationship with a given patient (see Chapter 5). Our ability to attune to our own emotional experience, verbalizable or not, must be a key instrument that we use as we attempt to promote in our patients awareness of and respect for the fullness of their emotional lives. Not only do we model such awareness and respect, we also use our emotional memory as a guide to optimal responsiveness. Thus clinical guidelines ought to be less precise and more general than they have traditionally been so that clinician's emotional knowledge can have room in which to work. Clinical supervision ought to support this use of affective memory and tacit knowledge to guide responsiveness in the treatment situation.

Not everyone agrees. Interpersonalist and social constructivist Donnel Stern (1989) writes of countertransference as our "unformulated experience" of patients. Like Sullivan (1940), he believes we must escape from the "grip" of the interpersonal field—the impasse created by the nonverbal experience of both people—by verbalization. Stern quotes Tauber and Green (1959) on respecting the grip of the field, noting that these authors believe that without the analyst's capacity to be so gripped, the patient "[would] have no respectable card of admission to the relationship" (p. 146, quoted in Donnel Stern, 1989, p. 21). Nevertheless, the grip must and can only be broken, according to Tauber and Green, by reflective verbalization.

Although Donnel Stern's "unformulated experience" may seem to resemble my concern for the tacit elements of experience, we have, I think, two differences. One concerns his belief that "it is only as experience can be verbally represented that it becomes valuable or informative" (p. 9). Without verbal articulation, we have only unformulated experience:

> Before being articulated the experiences are relatively undifferentiated, and thus in the sense that they cannot be known—cannot be reflected upon—they do not exist. Words do not clothe experience. They construct it. (1989, p. 1)

Donnel Stern assumes, unlike Polanyi, that knowledge requires differentiation and articulation. My conception of emotional memory, in contrast, intends to convey a positive regard for tacit knowledge as possessing its own truth and as sometimes diminished by our efforts to express it in words. (Nonliterary art forms such as dance express such an appreciation for the integrity of tacit knowing and a respect for what we sense.) Darlene Bregman Ehrenberg (1992) articulates the importance of tacit knowing and the limits of verbalization:

> It is well known that words can serve as barriers or bridges to communication, or as both simultaneously. Words can be used to conceal or reveal; they can be used in an attempt to evoke feelings or to elicit certain kinds of behavioral responses; they can be weapons, camouflage, cries for help, a means to test another, gifts, or even a way to put ideas and images into the mind of another. They can be used to seduce, amuse, amaze, charm, insult, penetrate, invade, betray, hurt, shock, deceive, distract, manipulate. . . . Since words can be a medium for acting out by patient or analyst, and since what goes on affectively, often nonverbally, can have profound impact, both positive and negative, the importance of becoming more aware of the impact of what goes on beyond words, even in the context of verbal communication, cannot be overestimated. (p. 14)

Second, some interpersonalists, and Donnel Stern in particular, seem to minimize the role of memory in shaping human experience and in the formation and maintenance of a sense of self. They speak as if analysis consists of horizontal slices of the here-and-now, in which only interpersonal influence in the present is examined. My view, like that of the developmental–relational theorists (e.g., Ghent, 1992), presupposes a longitudinal, developmental inquiry and sees the present as importantly formed by memory.

Even so, Donnel Stern calls attention to the centrality of the analyst's tacit experience of the patient. He suggests that gaining some access to this knowledge may break up therapeutic impasses. Such emphasis on the analyst's use of self-experience to understand relational experience, and vice versa, is one part of the pragmatic usefulness of the conception of emotional memory.

This chapter has investigated notions that we already use. Terms like the unconscious, sensorimotor knowledge, alexithymia, the prerepresentational self, and even affect have their place in historical and contemporary psychoanalytic discourse. Still, none of these quite captures the sense of visceral knowledge that I am calling "emotional memory." There may thus be a theoretical justification for coining a new term. My motivation, however, is more practical: The term "emotional memory" speaks to many patients with no translation and little explanation beyond saying that our history lives within us. I find that many patients use the term "emotional memory" as an access point to rich associative material.

The advantages also accrue to the analyst. If our theories use terms that need little translating, we can stay closer to the patient. In addition, using the term emotional memory encourages a salutary, intellectual humility. Technical terms can deceive us, and our patients, into thinking we know more than we do. If we have to say what we mean in everyday words, we are more likely to encounter the limits of our understanding, as well as the limits of the verbal realm. Perhaps as psychoanalytic fallibilists we will admit more often that we do not know very much. This more modest attitude can produce a "let's figure it out together" replacement for the psychoanalytic emphases on verbal interpretation as something an analyst gives to a patient and on the analyst's authority or expertise.

Finally, experience-near language is usually indefinite. Philosophers since Aristotle have cautioned us against seeking more precision than the subject at hand warrants. Emotional truth, powerful as it is, may often be uncertain as to content. As psychoanalysis gradually relinquishes its claim to be a natural science and takes its proper place among the realms of human wisdom, the uncertain and the imprecise will find the respect they deserve.

CHAPTER 9

Emotional Availability

> The quality of understanding is personally
> endured.
> —DINA VALLINO MACCIO, "Surviving,
> Existing, Living: Reflections on
> the Analyst's Anxiety"

*B*efore the emergence of the recent relational emphasis in psychoanalysis, analysts often attributed analytic success or failure to the "analyzability" of the patient. Now we place more weight on the abilities of a given analyst to work with a particular patient. We look at our emotional history and organizing principles, including our theories, and call these countertransference or cotransference (see Chapter 4), noting that they are often evoked by analytic work generally and by work with a particular analysand. In this chapter, however, I wish to consider a more general ability or disposition of analysts that I call "emotional availability." I view emotional availability as an underlying and often overlooked element in the success or failure of therapeutic relationships. It is an indispensable condition for the possibility of psychoanalytic understanding, and it thus deserves consideration as part of a psychoanalytic epistemology. Emotional availability is an active and responsive preparedness for empathic understanding.

Attachment researchers Emde and Sorce (1983) claim that the emotional availability of caretakers provides emotional security for infants and promotes their exploration in situations of uncertainty. By "emotional availability" they mean (1) the mother's communicating her awareness of the child's emotional states and (2) her readiness "to respond empathically and to offer her own emotional expressions as information when the infant is uncertain and looks to her" (p. 26). These researchers found that infants whose mothers were emotionally available showed more pleasure in play, a higher level of play, more exploration and curiosity, and more active—though less clingy—interest in their mothers than did those infants whose mothers were reading a newspaper. Emde and Sorce believe, thus, "that maternal emotional availability plays a crucial role in infant development since it helps to create an atmosphere that fosters enjoyment, curiosity, and enhanced opportunities for learning" (p. 28).

This view, reinforced by studies of infants with depressed caretakers (Cohn & Tronick, 1983; Tronick, 1989), has obvious implications for a developmental view of health and psychopathology. My concern here, however, is with a psychoanalytic parallel rather than with the developmental consequences of the argument made by Emde and Sorce. I think that the analyst's emotional availability provides an atmosphere of emotional safety that encourages exploration and curiosity in the patient in the same way that the caretaker's emotional availability does for the infant. In addition, I propose that emotional availability has the same components in both infancy and analysis and that it operates by the same primary communicative means, vocalization and visual referencing.

The first component of emotional availability is the caretaker's communication "through her behavior that she is aware of the infant's emotional expressions and is monitoring ongoing activity" (Emde & Sorce, 1983, p. 26). Similarly, Kohut (1971) pointed out the self-sustaining effects of parental mirroring of the child's emotional states. In analysis, we convey emotional availability to patients in various ways. We vocalize in verbal and semiverbal ways, fine-tuning our responses to convey our awareness of patients' emotional states by our choice of words and tone. We sit in ways that respond to patients' emotional communication, and we adjust the heating or lighting for their comfort. Once a patient decided to enter treatment with me because, she said, "You make faces." Whether or not I was saying anything, she could tell I was staying with her. For another person the "noises" I made performed a similar function, just as a listener on the telephone communicates attentiveness by making semiverbal sounds. Probably a person's inborn preference for visual or auditory processing combines with her or his emotional history to determine the channels of receptivity to emotional communications. Like sensitive parents, we must be ready to adjust our mode of expressing emotional availability to suit the receptive capacities of a particular patient.

This component of emotional availability, a readiness to attune and respond, is nonspecific. First, it can take many forms. We convey this readiness for attunement in many nonverbal ways, and thus it can be missed in written transcripts of treatment. A supervisor or consultant who looks for this intersubjectively determined capability for responsiveness may register its presence or absence in the supervisee's liking or disliking the patient. Its absence can also be detected in frequent distancing responses, often justified by reference to theories that support analytic neutrality and anonymity. Frequent reference to diagnostic categories is another indicator of emotional distancing. Embracing the concept of emotional availability erases neutrality and anonymity as rules for analytic conduct. Analysts who are emotionally available adjust how much they reveal of themselves to their patients to the needs of the individual patient, in the same way that parents attune their level of accessibility to the child.

This first component of emotional availability is nonspecific in another way. It is a general disposition, readiness, or responsiveness (Bacal, 1985), not a type of interpretation, intervention, or response. Lichtenberg, Lachmann, and Fosshage (1993) communicate this point by emphasizing the need to examine a sequence of analytic exchanges to gain a sense of the responsiveness of the analyst to the shifting and developing states and experiences of the patient. Emotional availability is captured beautifully in a photograph of Winnicott and a child patient (Grosskurth, 1987, p. 372). There he looks affectionately absorbed in and fascinated by the child, exemplifying his notion of "primary maternal preoccupation." In addition, his writings about infancy and about psychoanalysis, as well as Margaret Little's (1990) account of her analysis with him, convey Winnicott's awareness of the particular importance of his emotional availability in some treatments, especially those involving significant regression. Little's account further describes the interference of concurrent events in the analyst's life on his or her emotional availability and of the significant effects on treatment of even temporary unavailability of the analyst.

The Winnicottian "holding environment" is another way to speak of emotional availability. Its essential component—an attuned, nonintrusive presence—creates the emotional safety necessary for the development of a child's or patient's "true self" or "idiom" (Bollas, 1989). This nonspecific presence, or facilitating environment, makes possible the child's or patient's personal, idiosyncratic, and articulated selfhood.

Generality is another way to speak of the nonspecific character of emotional availability in both early caretakers and analysts. Many parents can respond only to those feelings and emotional expressions of their children that affirm themselves. Similarly, we analysts may have restrictions on our emotional responsiveness, overall or with some patients. One man, for example, remarked that his previous therapist was "all there" when he brought good news. When he was sad, disappointed, angry, or perplexed, she was "gone." Certain patients, moreover, come to us for just that generality of emotional availability that they miss in themselves. An actress once came into treatment with me because, she said, she could not "get into" some emotions and was thus restricted in the parts she could play well. Needing to find me emotionally available in just those areas where she was not, she was especially alert to my emotional limitations. Thus we analysts need to be aware of the limits of our potential for empathic responsiveness and work continuously to expand these abilities. Freud (1912) pointed toward this full availability of the analyst in his expression "evenly suspended attention" (p. 111). Unfortunately, he downplayed the emotional aspect both in this statement on technique and in his metaphor of the analyst as surgeon (1912, p. 115).

Let us now return to the definition of emotional availability provided by Emde and Sorce (1983): "She [the mother] is available to respond empathically and to offer her own emotional expressions as information when the infant is uncertain and looks to her" (p. 26). This readiness to offer our emotional expressions—verbal, semiverbal, or nonverbal—is a crucial component of the conversation that creates psychoanalytic understanding. We offer our emotional expressions, not as a substitute for those of the patient, but as pump-priming, or facilitating, responses, our participation in the analytic squiggle game (Winnicott, 1965). Often our attempts will be inaccurate, but in the atmosphere of emotional safety provided by this very responsiveness, many patients can use what we offer as a kind of catalyst for their own emotional expression. We show by such attempts that we are trying to understand, that we can imagine the patient to be having some emotional response, and that various—and perhaps less-than-elegant—expressions of emotion are more than acceptable to us. These attempts are trial balloons, similar to those interpretations by which we test the limits of our understanding (Winnicott, 1989), and they convey to the patient that guessing is just fine. Together we are attempting to find and create an understanding.

Concrete clinical expression of this emotional readiness to offer a response depends both on the therapist's style and on the intersubjective situation. With certain patients, I lean forward in my chair, and the conversation intensifies. Others are frightened by my leaning forward, and they lose track of what they were saying. With some patients, I start sessions by asking how they are feeling. This has the advantage of establishing an emotional communication from the beginning of the session. Often I respond quite spontaneously to stories I am told with "Oh, no!" or "Ouch!" With someone who finds it difficult to feel except by somatizing, I sometimes tell the patient what I or others have felt in similar situations. If I perceive that my trial balloon is not resonating with the patient, I will then ask again what the patient is feeling. My emotional responses and attempts to prime the pump often evoke emotion in patients, even in people generally distant from their emotional lives.

Reluctance to engage in such use of our own emotional life to get closer to patients and to support their expression and exploration may come from several sources. Many therapists endured the deprivation of a silent and invisible analyst who believed that this analytic posture would promote intrapsychic structuralization. Like parents who raise children as they were raised themselves, we often treat our patients as our analysts treated us. Another possibility is that some of us, like Freud, may dislike having others look at us for many hours a day. We may use the traditional analytic setup and procedures to protect ourselves from the effort of emotional engagement, which is so similar to the hard work of good-enough parenting. Too, we may be uncomfortable being wrong as much as we will inevitably be if we offer our emotional responses to patients, fearing that we may compromise our professional stature.

Another reasonable concern is our fear that our emotional availability will be experienced by the patients as intrusive, a fear that is especially likely if our own parents or analysts substituted their realities or agendas for ours. We must continuously monitor patients' experience of us, including their sense of our emotional response to them (Hoffman, 1983; Aron, 1991, 1992). This information provides a guide for when and how to offer our emotional responses. As with children, we see whether they feel free to come and go (as in secure attachment) or whether they become more than temporarily clingy or oppositional (as in insecure attachments). Emotional availability does not mean making or not making any particular response. Instead, it means a continuous readiness to explore thoughtfully the emotional experience, intersubjectively configured in the transference and cotransference, of whatever we do or do not do with the patient.

One young man had been seriously disorganized by the demands of his parents to adapt to their suddenly changing agendas. For the first 4 years of treatment he experienced almost anything I said or did as an attempt to crush him by imposing my thoughts, feelings, and needs on him. He used to complain that analysis and psychotherapy were set up, scheduled, and arranged for the convenience and needs of therapists and not of patients. After 4 years of treatment, he announced, "I think you are actually on my side." He had gradually come to see—by my having acknowledged and confirmed his view that my needs largely *did* structure the analytic situation—that I in fact accepted his sense of the tyranny of my interventions and of the whole arrangement. Feeling that his point of view had been accepted, he came to believe that I would seek and follow his agenda, which in time translated into a sense that I was with him, that I was emotionally available to support his growth into a person in his own right. In the words of Mitchell (1988):

> Unless the analyst affectively enters the patient's relational matrix or, rather, discovers himself within it—unless the analyst is in some sense charmed by the patient's entreaties, shaped by the patient's projec-

tions, antagonized and frustrated by the patient's defenses—the treatment is never fully engaged, and a certain depth within the analytic experience is lost. (p. 293)

Similarly Renik (1993) advocates revisions in our theory of technique "that will make it unnecessary for us to ask ourselves, in vain, not to be passionately and irrationally involved in our everyday clinical work" (p. 570).

In another instance of offering emotional expressions, I expressed a sense of differentness. A 40-year-old man who had devoted himself to improving the world through political action found himself isolated and depressed. He knew he had always felt this way, and he saw little hope for change in his experience. He came to each session saying he could not see what therapy was doing for him, or could do. He believed that only political and social changes were important; the minutiae of his feelings and history were uninteresting and mattered little. For months I tried to find ways to enter his experience and respond with empathic understanding. Finally I said that I had a different feeling, that, to me, the nuances, details, and "minutiae" of his emotional life and history *were* interesting and important, and that I guessed we really had a big difference of opinion. He left the session with a puzzled look. In his next session, however, he told me stories of his childhood, speculated about their influence on his life, and appeared genuinely interested in my comments. Although one could worry about compliance, this patient tends more to opposition. The change lasted, with some fits and starts. Perhaps, offering my interest—in Emde and Sorce's (1983) words, my emotional expressions—grounded him and gave him the emotional security needed for reflective exploration of his own experience.

A third fear related to offering patients our own emotional expressions is that it will make them dependent on us and will interfere with the articulated development of their own experience. Careful monitoring of the impact of our emotional availability on our patients can prevent this. Toddlers cling less and explore more when the caretaker is emotionally available but not intrusive. Many of our patients, however, come to us with seriously disturbed attachment histories. The most ordinary emotional availability or responsiveness, as Winnicott (1965) and Balint (1968) noted in their studies of regression to dependency, may evoke the response of a starving person when offered ordinary food. Or our patients may display the signs of the anxious, clingy attachment that a child would after a natural or human disaster. At this point, we therapists stand at an important intersection. We may panic in the face of the regression, ask ourselves what we are doing wrong, and then withdraw from the patient—perhaps by using a "borderline" diagnosis—confirming her or his worst fears. On the other hand, we can understand the clinging as a temporary traumatic response, remain emotionally available, and wait it out, trusting that emotional security will return or establish itself for the first time. We must know, even if the patient cannot, that dependency, within a secure attachment, is a necessary step on the road to the interdependence characteristic of mental health.

Finally, we may avoid emotional availability because it makes us feel vulnerable, not only to the patient but also to our own inevitably unfinished business. To understand from within emotional attachment means, as Ferenczi and others have found, that we revisit our own pain. I think that a principal reason for a training analysis is to know the sources of our own suffering deeply enough so that we can connect with the suffering of others. Knowing our cotransference—our personal history and our emotional organizing principles—can make greater emotional availability possible.

Two notes of caution are in order. The first is that emotional availability does not mean providing patients with whatever they want. The toddlers studied by Emde and Sorce were not allowed dangerous toys, and the mothers had to remain in their chairs. Parents must prevent children from doing dangerous things and from harming others. Similarly, we can set limits based on the needs of our patients or of our own. Like parents who need some rest or a moment to go to the bathroom, our emotional availability can have limits. Winnicott, for example, allowed himself to have a genuine vacation even if he had to hospitalize a patient to make this possible (Little, 1990). We must respond as fully as we can when we are with our patients and, like good parents, help them manage when we cannot be with them. Emotional availability, for analysts or for parents, does not mean having no limits or boundaries. It does, however, challenge us to understand where and why we set these limits.

Second, emotional availability is always limited by the particularity of analyst and patient. Our cotransference includes our emotional history and the general inferences (organizing principles) we have drawn about ourselves and others from this history. These principles lead us to adopt theories of human nature, some of which may be psychoanalytic theories. These theories also form part of our cotransference, and they limit or expand our emotional availability to patients generally. This is particularly evident with patients whose emotional organization interacts with ours, making us more or less or differently responsive.

Many impasses in treatment develop because the organizing principles of patient and analyst are too different for them to find or maintain a common ground of understanding. Other treatment problems develop, as the intersubjectivity theorists have repeatedly shown (Stolorow et al., 1987), because analyst and patient are too similar in their emotional organization. This situation, or "intersubjective conjunction," can make it difficult to recognize what is going wrong, or why the treatment seems not to be progressing. A 40-year-old woman, for example, came for treatment because of intense anxiety and growing depression, with an alarming wish to be dead that she related to her failing marriage. She had, out of deference to her parents' wishes, married a wealthy man and had become a very competent servant, managing the home and providing excellent care for their two daughters, now adolescents. She reminded me of Stevens, the butler in *Remains of the Day*. With no sense of a life, or preferences, or opinions, or purposes of her own, her only function was to make sure things ran smoothly for the nuclear and extended families. In the culture of both her and her husband's families, this was the only role for a woman, even an extremely intelligent one.

For many years, by her original account, the system had run smoothly. Her family of origin had been "wonderful" and her marriage "okay." Only now, when she had developed a friendship with another married woman, had she begun to feel so anxious and depressed. The company of this friend made her feel important in her own right, and comfortable and safe in ways she could never remember having felt before. Within this context, she began to realize what she had been missing. In addition, the contrast between her marriage and that of her friend brought despair over her own future life prospects and anxiety at the almost inconceivable thought of her own freedom. She preferred not to discuss the loneliness of her own marriage, nor the anger she sometimes momentarily felt when her husband berated her or failed to volunteer any help at times when she was obviously overburdened. What she wanted from me was help with feeling better, putting options out of her mind, and putting up with the conditions of her life.

My original sense was that I was very different from her. She seemed to feel entirely trapped while I had, after all, left a destructive marriage. If she could just come to understand what I had come to understand and feel, she could be just fine. I, of course, knew what would be best for her. The intersubjective field formed by my agenda and sense of things—undoubtedly indirectly communicated—with her very strong tendency to comply with others' expectations of her only heightened her anxiety. Torn among complying with her parents' expectations, her husband's demands, and now my agenda, she felt bound to lose someone. For all sorts of "practical" reasons, she became unable to keep regular appointments. The needs of others always intervened.

Realizing that the treatment was failing, I had to enlarge my perspective. In order to do this, I needed to become aware of my own emotional organizing principles and needs, to see how similar these were to hers and to recognize my own impact on the treatment. What helped me was noticing this patient's ways of taking care of me in sessions—telling me she was fine, asking about my well-being, watching the clock—and remembering how I had been like that with my own analyst. This patient and I were very alike in our compulsive caretaking and in our assumption that our only value as persons lay in our capacity and skill as caretakers. So I was taking care of her, trying to fix her life—in proper analytic interpretive style, of course—and she was taking care of me, trying to establish her value in my eyes and to maintain her fragile sense of worth in her own eyes.

When we reflected together on our caretaking patterns, changes began. The need to be helpful and caretaking loosened its grip on me, and her freedom in relation to me very gradually increased. Our tie no longer depended on her divining and complying with my hopes for her. We began to talk more about the complexity of compliance, caretaking, and the loss of selfhood required to maintain ties in her family of origin and in her current family. I began to be more able to feel my way into her emotional predicament. Simultaneously she began to report more sustained frustration with her marriage and her family role, along with some efforts to tell her husband and children that she expected respectful treatment. She also began to ask them for occasional help, and she was surprised that they protested less than she had expected. She is working at perceiving and following her own feelings and interests, and she is just beginning to sense that these will lead her wherever she needs to go. As a result, she feels less trapped. She does feel a new kind of sadness—less despairing, but full of mourning for the person she never had a chance to become.

This story illustrates the need to be aware of the inevitable cotransferential limits on our emotional availability to patients. Such discoveries led Ferenczi to his experiments in mutual analysis. At the very least we need self-reflection and consultation to maintain and develop our emotional availability.

In conclusion, emotional availability provides needed balance in the mutual but asymmetrical (Aron, 1992) analytic relationship. Long ago Aristotle (*Nicomachean Ethics*) noted that friendship requires some sort of equality between the friends. In analysis or in analytic psychotherapies, the educated emotional availability that the analyst can offer balances the money and vulnerability that patients must provide. This is an asymmetry patients often find so shameful that they call it "paid friendship." We must acknowledge some truth in their complaint, but also ask if our distancing makes the asymmetry more painful than necessary. Some writers (e.g., Hoffman, 1993) speak of the analyst's authority or expertise. I suggest that if the analyst is an expert, this expertise consists primarily in a capacity, probably both innate and learned, for reflective emotional availability.

BETTER LATE THAN NEVER: THE EMOTIONALLY AVAILABLE WITNESS

Emotional availability, an idea borrowed from attachment theory (Emde & Sorce, 1983), fits easily into my view of self psychology.

Serving selfobject functions, or providing opportunities for selfobject experience, requires emotional availability. Here let us examine a form of selfobject experience particularly important in the treatment of trauma survivors, the special emotional ability or readiness of the analyst or therapist to be a witness.

Self psychology has, from its inception, identified the mirroring of a child's natural grandiosity or expansiveness as an essential ingredient of healthy development. It has named this mirroring "selfobject" responsiveness to indicate that a child, or anyone, can use mirroring to build and maintain a continuous, cohesive, and positively valued sense of self. Here I wish to draw attention to another selfobject experience—closely related to mirroring—particularly involved in psychoanalytic healing. For now let us agree to call this the "selfobject experience of witness." Witnessing, a special form of participation in the intersubjective field, makes the other's experience real and valid and important to that other.

In *The Untouched Key: Tracing Childhood Trauma in Creativity and Destructiveness,* Alice Miller (1990) claims that the crucial difference in the outcome of severe child abuse depends on the presence of someone in the child's life who witnesses, and thus gives the child the opportunity and ability to experience, the child's pain. Without such a witness, Miller believes, the child cannot experience the abuse as abuse. Instead it is torture that must be endured. The child often feels she or he deserves treatment that an observer would see as cruel and outrageous. In the presence of some, even minimally, validating witness, the child can experience the abuse as mistreatment and, thereby, find ways to express it, perhaps in art. In Miller's words:

> Men of various professions frequently ask me why they didn't become a Hitler but have lived their lives as more or less peaceful physicians, lawyers, or professors, even though they, like Hitler, were beaten every day when they were children. They use this question to argue against my thesis that brutal, unfeeling, and thoroughly destructive treatment of children produces monsters—not by chance but of necessity. Then I always inquire about the details of the person's childhood, and on closer examination it turns out in every case that a particular witness helped the child experience his feelings to some degree. In Adolf Hitler's childhood, such a stabilizing witness was totally lacking. I have often compared the structure of

Hitler's family to a totalitarian regime in which there is no possibility of recourse against the police state. (pp. 50–51)

In treatment, we can often find that there was a witness in the patient's history, however occasional and fleeting. Indeed, the existence of such a witness may be a necessary precondition for the possibility of seeking treatment, that is, for at least minimal hope that a human being or a human connection can help. We find, nevertheless, that many patients with severe self disturbances are able to find in treatment, apparently for the first time, just such a witness. Miller, in fact, applies her theory to the treatment of children:

> If mistreated children are not to become criminals or mentally ill, it is essential that *at least once in their life* they come in contact with a person who knows without any doubt that the environment, not the helpless, battered child, is at fault. . . . Here lies the great opportunity for relatives, social workers, therapists, teachers, doctors, psychiatrists, officials and nurses *to support the child and to believe her or him.* (pp. 168–169)

Similarly, the analyst or therapist who wants to understand what happened to the child whose adult self comes for treatment becomes the witness who makes it possible for the adult to experience the full horror of his or her history, and thus to begin to heal. What we often call denial, disavowal, or unconsciousness may often be experience never truly experienced (cf. Stolorow & Atwood, 1992). It may be the given (the brute event) of which we can make (construe, organize) nothing. When patients tell us that no one but the analyst understands, they often mean that they are only beginning to know their history. Such clinical phenomena point to the thoroughly intersubjective character of self-knowledge.

The following examples illustrate the therapeutic function of witnessing: Consider Terry, the patient of mine described in Chapter 8, "Emotional Memory."[*] Her father's family has a complex history of incest (family members are often related both as child and sibling, for example) and violence—her father had mur-

---

[*]The description of Terry's history to follow is different from the one in Chapter 8 because it includes information recalled later in the analysis.

dered someone, and for many years he beat and raped his wife, daughters, and son. Her mother's family is also violent and continues to practice revengeful sorcery.

Her mother's continuing denial, her inability to be a witness, exacerbates Terry's struggle to reclaim her history, and thus herself. This patient, in her mid-20s, exhibits the severe discontinuities of self-experience typical of multiple personalities. (Many cases of discontinuity in self- experience—psychiatry calls these dissociative phenomena—may result from the absence, at crucial moments in a person's history, of the validating witness.) The flashbacks Terry suffers in treatment allow me to serve as a witness, and this, in turn, enables Terry to establish the continuity of her experience. My emotional availability has been necessary to produce enough of a sense of safety and of self-cohesion to make it possible for Terry to recognize her terrors as memory.

Another patient, Cheryl, is the child of parents who are disturbed in various impulsive and narcissistic ways. On the surface, Cheryl appears to have every advantage—she is strikingly good-looking, highly intelligent, and affluent. Initially Cheryl could not understand why she was so anxious and depressed. After our extensive work at making sense together of her subjective experience, she began to empathize with her emotional life and find it valid. In her words, "I see that there are reasons for my feelings." Once she found that she could use me as a witness to her painful history, thereby becoming able to possess and articulate her experience, she began to find witnesses and soulmates in literature. She would bring examples into the treatment. "Have you ever read *The Man Without a Country*?" she asked. "I feel just like the person who belongs nowhere and to nobody." She then found similar selfobject experiences in the human world outside treatment.

For such patients defense and resistance protect a vulnerable self from retraumatization. Remembering is experienced as dangerous partly because it includes the memory of being alone with whatever the trouble was, without the support and validation of witness. Not until the tie to the analyst is strong can vivid kinds of remembering be risked, for without a secure connection the patient's fear that the memories will be overwhelming and lead to psychosis or self-destruction prevents their emergence. The tie to the analyst makes it possible for the patient to discover and to survive realizing—making real—the full horror of what happened to her or him as a vulnerable child. Part of the horror was being alone.

Clinical experience leads me to speculate that for those patients who had someone to be a witness, and the more reliable that witness remained for them, the sooner such a memory-permitting tie to the analyst becomes possible. In contrast to Terry, Sara, the daughter of an alcoholic father and a psychotically depressed mother, had a first-grade teacher whose home she and a sibling visited every day after school for their remaining school years. This patient had no memory of having discussed being berated, beaten, locked in basements, and, much less, molested, with this teacher. She was unsure whether the teacher was aware of her home situation. Still, "she never sent us home, and never asked why we came over so much." In treatment, this patient did exhibit severe "dread to repeat" what had happened to her, the phenomenon described by A. Ornstein (1991). This dread was most evident in a hyperalertness to, and curiosity about, my thoughts and reactions. Such caution and attunement had been an indispensable protection from violence in her childhood. Still, her readiness to use me as a witness, demonstrated by the early and steady availability of traumatic memories, is most likely due in part to the selfobject function of witnessing provided by Sara's teacher. When prolonged misunderstandings occur between us, however, Sara begins to feel that she remembers little or nothing of her childhood. When her sense of my availability as a witness is restored, she resumes the process of coming to know her own history.

The notion of an emotionally available witness offers an intersubjective account of the analyst's contribution to the process of remembering. It allows us to describe a selfobject process in which previously unavailable history becomes experience that contributes to self-consolidation. History becomes self-experience, becomes "my history," in the presence of the other who says, in one way or another, "That is horrible. That should never happen to a child."

This witnessing is indeed a subset of mirroring if mirroring means appreciative response to what is valuable in the child. Implicitly it says to the person, "I see you as precious and worthy of respectful treatment. You had no way to know the horror of what happened to you because you were treated as worthless or bad." Witnessing is also part of the validation that makes possible the child's trust in her or his own experience and sense of the real. This thoroughly intersubjective conception assumes the need for the other as a condition for the very possibility of experience. According to Stolorow and Atwood (1992), "the child's conscious experience becomes progressively *articulated* through the validating responsiveness of the early surround" (p. 31). Both the appreciative responsiveness of mirroring and the confirming responsiveness of validation are involved in witnessing. The specificity of witnessing is the recognition of the horror, of the mistreatment, of the pain that otherwise cannot become fully conscious experience. The pain is brutally given, relatively unorganized experience. It needs the responsive emotionality of the intersubjective field or potential space (Winnicott, 1971) to allow it to become real and meaningful experience. The patient, in other words, can experience raw pain but needs the responsive other to construe it, to understand its enormity and meaning. Analyst and patient make sense of it together.

To recapitulate, witnessing means the presence of a responsive person who makes it possible for the child, or a patient who was the child, to recognize the horror of whatever happened to him or her and to feel the appropriate pain. Witnessing allows the child to experience and the patient to remember. It thus undoes dissociation and allows a person to establish the continuity of a self-possessed life. It undoes shame and restores the positive valuation of the self. It establishes and maintains self-experience, and it clearly deserves designation as a "selfobject" function. In cases of posttraumatic stress, witnessing is one form the emotional availability of the analyst must take.

Emotional availability is an essential practical condition for making sense together and for the possibility of a developmental second chance in psychoanalysis. With good theory held lightly, and emotional availability offered generously, a clinician has the fundamentals for psychoanalytic understanding.

CHAPTER 10

Misunderstanding: A Collaborative- Pragmatist View

I am the master of this college, and what I
know not, is not knowledge.
                —Attributed to WILLIAM WHEWELL,
                                of Oxford

Pragmatism unstiffens all our theories.
                —WILLIAM JAMES, *Pragmatism*

*M*isunderstanding is not the logical opposite to understanding. Instead, misunderstanding is inherent in the process of understanding, and it is often the normal condition of psychoanalytic work. Infant research has shown that attunement requires continual mutual readjustment between mother and infant (Daniel Stern, 1985; Beebe & Lachmann, 1994). Self psychology has highlighted the constructive potential of empathic disjunctions or ruptures. Misunderstanding and lack of understanding in the clinical situation can lead to deeper and fuller understanding, including more intimate mutual attachment. In Kohut's (1994) words, "The long not-being-able-to-understand is often the necessary precondition for a deeper understanding" (p. 264). Such a view, however, requires a rethinking of ordinary either–or views of truth and reality, and it implies a pragmatist's commitment to a thoroughgoing philosophical fallibilism. Unnecessary misunderstanding can result from theoretical inflexibility and dogma. The collaborative pragmatist, on the contrary, works with the patient to make sense of emotional experience.

TRUTH AND REALITY IN PSYCHOANALYSIS

Psychoanalytic understanding clearly has something to do with truth and reality. The nature of truth and reality, however, is not so clear. One approach is to shrug our shoulders and concede that philosophers have been struggling to find adequate conceptions of truth and reality for millennia now.Surely we psychoanalysts ought not to expect to find an easy resolution to this quandary. But we cannot ignore the issue of the nature of truth and reality because it has practical bearings on psychoanalytic theory (according to James, 1907, there is nothing so practical as a good theory) and on our clinical work.

Let us address theory first. If we view understanding as intentional (in the phenomenological sense, that is, as understanding of *something*), then we immediately confront the twin issues of epistemology and ontology. Epistemology focuses on the question of the adequacy (or truth) of our understanding; ontology addresses the status (real or imaginary?) of whatever we seek to understand—a thing, a text, a person, an idea, or logical statement. Psychoanalytic epistemology raises these same questions. We ask both how well we understand (epistemology), and also what level of reality we are meeting ("I'd like to wring her neck" vs. "I plan to shoot her tonight"). If we fail to reflect on these philosophical issues, we doom ourselves to the psychoanalytic unexamined life. Those who eschew metaphysics, goes the old philosophical saw, will be controlled by unconscious metaphysics. I do not attempt a Kleinian (G. Klein, 1976) "theorectomy" or, what is similar, a Husserlian cleansing of presuppositions. Instead, I suggest that we psychoanalytic theoreticians make our unconscious philosophical presuppositions—about knowing, reality, and human nature and motivation, for example—as conscious as we can. Only then can these intellectual organizing principles leave the closed Cartesian study for the open smoke-free rooms of dialogue.

On the practical and clinical side, unexamined conceptions of truth and reality can wreak havoc. They contribute to many serious instances of misunderstanding. Most therapists are likely to have worked with patients who have lost trust in themselves or in the possibility of therapeutic help because, in the name of truth or reality, previous therapists have undermined or invalidated the patients' sense of things. Clinical use of conceptions like transference as distortion, can mean to the patient that the analyst possesses truth or reality, and that the patient does not. Of course, therapists hope that patients do not lose faith in themselves as a result of having been in therapy. Such misunderstandings—often the result of our theoretical and practical choice of position—are unproductive and should occur infrequently in a psychoanalysis conducted in a collaborative (making sense together) and fallibilist spirit.

I propose, therefore, to review some major conceptions of truth and reality in modern philosophy and in the history of psychoanalysis. I will then articulate some conceptions of truth and reality most consistent with an intersubjective view of psychoanalytic understanding.

The venerable philosophical question of the nature of truth has become a major issue in psychoanalysis today, probably to the advantage of both disciplines. Philosophy may clarify its old questions by seeing them worked out in a newer venue. Psychoanalysis stands to gain a clearer understanding of its own premises, especially of its devotion to reflective awareness.

Correspondence Theories of Truth

Most psychoanalysts discuss the nature of truth as if two, and only two, options existed. The first is the common sense theory, also known as the correspondence theory of truth. In philosophy the precursors of this approach are Locke and Hume, and its ordinary guise is the ontology of naive realism. According to correspondence theories, ideas in the mind are more or less accurate copies of things, facts, realities, or states of affairs that exist; the existence of these is not dependent on whether humans have any knowledge or awareness of them (Potter, 1994). Truth exists when ideas match, or correspond to, external realities, when language accurately pictures the world (Wittgenstein, 1921). The conceptual problems with this point of view appear when we consider how to test the match tetween ideas and those external realities. In a sense we need to introduce another mind (an outside authority), to judge, and the accuracy of this judge in turn requires checking, and so on to infinite regress. The ideas we are trying to match to external reality we arrive at by necessarily subjective means ("To me, my father was a giant"). The requirement by correspondence theories that subjectively derived ideas be "objectively" verified ends up reducing subjectivity's usefulness to that of a more or less competent copy machine. This reduction eliminates the only matter of interest to psychoanalysis or accessible to psychoanalytic inquiry—the experience of the subject.

Nevertheless, correspondence theories were much in vogue when psychoanalysis was born in the late 19th and early 20th centuries. Logical positivism—the intellectual offspring of the successes of modern science—produced the verification criterion for evaluating scientific theories. According to logical positivists, a theory is only as good as the quantifiable experimental evidence that supports or verifies it. In a weaker form,* positivism views theoretical statements as bearing meaning or cognitive significance only to the extent that their proponents can specify what experimental evidence would count as falsifying the theory. Either way, for the logical positivist truth is the match between theory and experimental evidence.

In psychoanalysis, correspondence theorists are most identifiable by their devotion to the idea of transference as distortion, the mismatch between a patient's sense of things and the analyst's "reality." Correspondence theorists also tend to object strenuously to the narrative-truth views of Spence and Schafer. Charles Hanly (1992), a psychoanalyst who calls his view "scientific realism," recently endorsed a correspondence theory. Likewise, interpersonalist Zucker (1993), in "Reality: Can It Be Only Yours or Mine?" asserts:

---

*Positivists consider it easier to falsify a theory than to verify it. One good counterexample, in this view, disproves a theory.

The problem of establishing well-grounded knowledge in our field is exceedingly difficult, but this is no warrant for surrendering to the lures of subjectivity. Our field has hardly addressed itself to developing methodologies equal to the difficulty and complexity of our material. It has done little, if anything, on such problems as what constitutes data, what is the potential of different kinds of data for activating experience, it commonly mistakes abstractions for raw data, it has not worked on, let alone developed rules of evidence in relation to data and, in my opinion, has not required and trained for a high standard of reasoning and logic in its thinking. (p. 485)

Zucker apparently believes that psychoanalytic data can be evaluated on other than subjective grounds. Although psychoanalysis surely involves some quantifiable aspects appropriate for empirical research, I believe with Kohut (1959) that only the study of data obtained by introspection and empathy is truly psychoanalytic. To know anything thoroughly is to surrender to its lure, and to know anyone psychoanalytically we must surrender to the lure of subjectivity. Zucker's experience-distant logic, the logic of empiricism and positivism, tests theoretical ideas against "the facts"—which positivism believes to be independent of observer bias—and checks to see whether theory and fact match up. On the contrary, clinical and theoretical reasoning in psychoanalysis, like the scientific logic of discovery, must remain close to experience. In the logic of discovery, the important work is the collaborative framing of plausible hypotheses or surmises (making sense together) to account for surprises or anomalies. We do need this kind of logic in psychoanalysis. It will allow us to take subjective experience seriously, and still do justice to the common sense embedded in correspondence theories.

Coherence Theories of Truth

While correspondence theories define truth as factual accuracy, coherence theories—the second approach to the nature of truth—define truth as what "rings true," a reference to subjectivity. Coherence theories, emphasizing the unavoidable contribution of the human mind to all knowing, highlight the limits of knowledge. Proponents of coherence theories claim, modestly and accurately in their opinion, that truth exists to the extent to which ideas hang together, or cohere. To decide truth and falsehood, they consider logical criteria such as consistency, elegance (i.e., parsimony), and the absence of internal contradiction. Coherence theorists count Kant and Hegel among their philosophical ancestors. In this century, the hermeneutics of Gadamer and the postempiricist philosophies of science of Kuhn and Feyerabend are well-known representatives of the coherence theory of truth. Prominent psychoanalytic advocates of this point of view include Spence (1982), Schafer (1983), Hoffman (1991), and, in self psychology, Goldberg (1988).

The correspondence and coherence theories of truth are more or less practical methods for evaluating the worth of ideas. Yet we can also see that they bear on our modes of relating. Empiricist theories fit most naturally with critical and competitive modes of relating. Coherence theories usually assume that we find truth through collaboration and thus bear a closer resemblance to the pragmatist ideas to be considered next.

The Pragmatist Shift to Meaning

In ordinary life, the kind we live when we are less aware of being philosophers or psychoanalysts, we use both theories. I use an almost automatic correspondence theory to check whether my idea that I turned off the stove matches the dials and lights on the stove itself. Analogously, if I sit on a jury in a trial where physical evidence is scarce, I use a coherence theory of truth to evaluate the stories I hear. Both approaches to evaluating ideas function in our everyday thinking. Further, each method has yielded a theory of truth that its adherents claim is the ultimate truth about truth. Nevertheless, neither theory alone is a good-enough theory to account for daily experience. We need to seek a more adequate or comprehensive theory of truth.

Fortunately, we have a third opinion, which has sources in American philosophy and deeper roots in Aristotle and Kant. This view is the pragmatist shift from truth to meaning. William James (1907) described this shift with his usual charm:

> I am happy to say that it is the English-speaking philosophers who first introduced the custom of interpreting the meaning of concep-

tions by asking what difference they make for life. Mr. Peirce has only expressed in the form of an explicit maxim what their sense for reality led them all instinctively to do. The great English way of investigating a conception is to ask yourself right off, "What is it *known as?*" In what facts does it result? What is its *cash-value,* in terms of particular experience? And what special difference would come into the world according as it were true or false? (p. 268)

Peirce (1877) provided the more precise maxim to which James referred:

> Consider what effects, that might *conceivably* have practical bearings, we *conceive* the object of our *conception* to have. Then, our *conception* of these effects is the whole of our *conception* of the object. (vol. 5, p. 258)

Thus practical bearings and intellectual conceptions were, for Peirce, inextricably linked, perhaps differing only as foreground and background do in Gestalt studies. Both James and Peirce made the shift in theory, so natural in practice for psychoanalysts, to a pragmatic, or meaning-based, view of the nature of truth. Both were asking not for truth itself but for the difference it makes in the conduct of life to think one way or another. Peirce (1877) elaborated:

> The whole function of thought is to produce habits of action; and . . . whatever there is connected with a thought, but irrelevant to its purpose, is an accretion to it, but no part of it. If there be a unity among our sensations which has no reference to how we shall act on a given occasion, as when we listen to a piece of music, why we do not call that thinking. To develop its meaning, we have, therefore, simply to determine what habits it produces, for what a thing means is simply what habits it involves. Now, the identity of a habit depends on how it might lead us to act, not merely under such circumstances as are likely to arise, but under such as might possibly occur, no matter how improbable they may be. What the habit is depends on *when* and *how* it causes us to act. . . . Thus, we come down to what is tangible and conceivably practical, as the root of every real distinction of thought, no matter how subtle it may be; and there is no distinction of meaning so fine as to consist in anything but a possible difference of practice. (vol. 5, pp. 256–257)

MEANING AND PSYCHOANALYTIC UNDERSTANDING

A shift to a focus on meaning has many logical corollaries, equivalent for a pragmatist to practical consequences. The remainder of this chapter will address those practical consequences for understanding and misunderstanding in psychoanalysis.

The first of the corollaries is that both popular theories of truth—the correspondence and coherence theories—are inadequate. To assess the truth of our ideas, we need the reference to the external world, the point of reference central to the correspondence theories. We also require the reference to conceptual unity, which is basic to the coherence theories. Nevertheless, the two approaches do not add up to the whole truth; taken separately or together, they reduce truth to a sort of solution to a puzzle. They remove truth from the realm of human experience and of temporal and historical process. Only a shift to a pragmatic, or meaning-based, conception of truth can overcome these problems.

In psychoanalysis, similarly, we can see that each traditional theory of truth is a partial truth. A psychoanalyst announces to her patients a planned week of vacation. One patient says the analyst is selfish and thinks only of herself. If the analyst really understood, and took seriously, the patient's suffering, she would not leave. A second patient envies the analyst, seeing her as rich, privileged, and free to pursue her pleasures. Another believes the analyst must be ill or on the verge of burnout. A fourth says, well, everybody takes vacations—have a good time. The next is convinced that either patient or analyst will die or come to harm during the vacation. Neither a correspondence view ("No, you're wrong"), nor a coherence response ("Well, does that fit with what else you know about me?" or "I guess this fits with what we know about *you*!") will help here.

Such a common clinical situation illustrates the need for a pragmatic, or meaning-oriented theory of truth. The correctness or falsehood of patient beliefs about the vacation is trivial compared with the immense importance of their meaning, or practical bearing, for the patient. These meanings are distinct exactly insofar as they affect the patient's habits of action and interpretation, the analyst's response to the patient's interpretations, and thus the intersubjective field of the analysis. The shift to meaning does not imply that we gain access to "the whole truth," but rather improves the likelihood that we are considering some kind of truth that matters.

The second corollary of a pragmatic theory is that our psychoanalytic theories differ in meaning only to the extent that they lead us to different habitual responses to patients. Believers in the principle of distortion—most Freudian and Kleinian analysts—will pursue some line of interpretation designed to convince the patient that instinctual wishes and fantasies determine and distort his or her responses. Self psychologists may say that each patient response expresses the real state of the selfobject experience, and the therapist will respond with that specific understanding. A collaborative pragmatist may, depending on the situation, simply accept the patient's view. Then she or he will work collaboratively with the patient to figure out the meanings of the vacation, of the way it was announced, of the patient's response, and of its effect on the joint psychoanalytic experience.

Our theories of truth also bear on the question of theory-choice (see Chapter 3). We choose theories (engage in theory-choice) neither for their correspondence properties, which we can never adequately check, nor simply for their elegant wholeness. Instead, in a fallibilist and pragmatist spirit, we embrace them for the help they provide in elucidating meanings in practical ways and for shaping our responses to situations we have not yet envisioned. We can now see more clearly that a psychoanalytic theory is more than a conceptual scheme. It is a way of being with people, a way of life.

A third corollary of the shift to a focus on meaning is fallibilism, the systematic and persistent recognition that one can always be mistaken. Fallibilism acknowledges the inevitable limits on any individual's, or any finite number of individuals', ability to know. It replaces the search for certainty and distortion-correction with a dialogic search for reasonableness or meaning in a community of inquirers. In the psychoanalytic situation, fallibilism means the assumption that understanding is always partial, incomplete, and capable of improvement. Fallibilism is an intrinsic facet of a pragmatic approach to the search for truth and meaning, and of the perspectival realism (see Chapter 4) that matches it in ontology.

In the psychoanalytic situation, the analyst's fallibilism can produce, or at least make possible, greater patient self-reflectiveness. The analysis becomes a safe place to come to know and remember who one is and what makes one tick. Theoretical fallibilism can engender a collaborative "let's figure this out together" atmosphere, one in which it feels safer to wonder, to do thought experiments and feeling experiments in the transference with a trusted guide and companion. Some sorts of defensiveness and resistance may never appear in such an analysis (Brandchaft, 1983), and other forms of self-protectiveness may become superfluous over time. Hoffman (1987) describes some of the advantages of adopting an attitude of theoretical fallibilism in his article "The Value of Uncertainty in Psychoanalytic Practice."

To read, however, recent discussions of what analysts' authority and expertise should be is to wonder whether we truly see ourselves as collaborators and participants on the side of the patient's emerging selfhood in a struggle for meaning and truth. Perhaps instead we still seek some correspondence- or coherence-based certainty. Tansey (1992), for example, has compared conceptions of analytic expertise in what Mitchell (1988) calls the drive-conflict, developmental arrest, and relational-conflict models. Tansey prefers the relational-conflict model, which "calls upon the analyst to be expert at generating collaborative inquiry with the patient into repetitive patterns of interaction as they unfold within the treatment relationship in one form or another" (p. 314). In addition to questioning the original classification (I believe that one can be a developmentalist without allegiance to a simplistic developmental arrest model), as a fallibilist I have additional questions. Why is it so important to assert our expertise, even if its nature is as benign as the sort Tansey attributes to the relational-conflict theorist? If his aim is the reduction of the extreme relational asymmetry he finds in the other models, then why concentrate on expertise at all? What are we afraid of losing?

Similarly, Hoffman's (1993) treatment of "the intimate authority of the psychoanalyst's presence" presents a collaborative picture of the analytic relationship. Still, if authority and power are so important, isn't the patient an authority and an expert on her or his own life? Why are our authority and expertise so important to us? Usually when people feel adequately confident—even if that confidence includes appropriate uncertainty about what they are doing—they feel no need to emphasize their authority, power, and expertise. When analysts can live with uncertainty, they provide a space for the process of understanding and avoid the rigidity that contributes to unnecessary misunderstandings.

CLINICAL THEORY AS A SOURCE OF MISUNDERSTANDING

The search for certainty, however, is not the only source of misunderstanding in psychoanalysis. Analysts' attachment to metapsychologies and their associated clinical theories can contribute to many an impasse. Momentarily bypassing other sources of analysts' cotransference, this section will provide an example of the influence of our clinical theories on misunderstanding in analytic work. We can no longer regard the patient as the sole source of trouble; misunderstanding is a thoroughly intersubjective phenomenon (Brandchaft, 1985). Patients bring to the field of the psychoanalytic encounter their emotional history, their dreads and longings, and their patterned ways of responding and of organizing emotional experience. We analysts and therapists bring all these same influences, plus general and clinical theories. The illustration to follow is one of many possible examples. Other influences would include clinical theories based on mechanistic metapsychologies, ethnocentrism, sexist assumptions, homophobia, and the equation of schizophrenic autistic states with normal infancy.

The misunderstanding I will focus on results, I believe, from an overreliance on the traditional psychoanalytic conception of object constancy. I will briefly present some recent history of the concept of object constancy and then elaborate my concern about both its theoretical underpinnings and its application in clinical situations.

As the term is generally used, "object constancy" denotes the developmental achievement of the ability to retain an image or representation of the caretaker in her or his absence. Debate about when this can be accomplished usually turns on the question of when infants possess or develop particular cognitive capacities and on how such capacities may be related to the achievement of object constancy. Those, for example, who regard Piagetian object permanence as a prerequisite for object constancy will place its achievement later than do those who do not. Whenever object constancy is achieved, what is ordinarily thought to be at stake is libidinal object constancy, the ability to regard the object as reliably existent whether it is felt as gratifying (present) or frustrating (absent). This capacity is supposed to overcome, or preclude the need for, such early defenses as splitting and denial. In the view of Mahler, Pine, and Bergman (1975), object constancy makes possible a healthy resolution of the separation–individuation process.

Proponents of this view see the absence of object constancy in adult life and in treatment as primarily attributable to an excess of constitutional aggression. Such a lack, they believe, paradoxically results in excessive expression of instinctual drives, as well as in early and sometimes unstable defensive systems, leading in treatment to chaotic transference reactions. This theory blames the failure to achieve libidinal object constancy for "borderline" behavior and personality organization.

There are theoretical problems in this formulation. It relies on a biological and drive-based, not an experience-based, conception of human motivation. In addition, it depends on an intrapsychic, or one-person, idea of development. It deemphasizes the relational context or intersubjective field, so we find little reference to parental consistency as a developmental influence on the child's ability to experience the parent as a constant object. Similarly, this view overlooks the question of the therapist's consistency of responsiveness in what appears to be a patient's lack of object constancy. What we need is a thoroughly intersubjective understanding of how children develop the ability to retain a sense of connection to their caretakers and, analogously, of how this process unfolds in an analysis.

Above all, I suspect that the emphasis on the lack of libidinal object constancy often misses the importance of the reverse phenomenon, the importance to the child or patient of the sense of being held in memory by the caretaker or therapist, of existing with constancy for the other. Perhaps the capacity to feel remembered by another, or to feel continuously significant for the other, is a usually taken-for-granted prerequisite for being able to benefit from the particular selfobject process sometimes called a "holding environment" (Winnicott, 1965). This capacity, which may be a basic condition for the possibility of many selfobject experiences, allows a person to feel continuously and stably existing for another, or perhaps even significant to the other. Such a capacity is not a quality of an isolated mind (Stolorow & Atwood, 1992); its development requires the presence of a stable and attentive other. Its absence usually suggests serious disruptions in early attachment experiences. The therapist's ability to hold the patient in memory and to express this holding—another form of emotional availability—together with the patient's gradually attained capacity to experience, and to rely on, being held in memory, may then make possible other developmental processes.

In treatment, some patients seem to have enormous difficulty feeling remembered by their therapist or analyst. Once we bring this difficulty to the foreground of our awareness, we can notice a range of clinical phenomena. The most extreme examples, and those that have alerted me to this difficulty, involve patients who feel nonexistent and become panicky when they cannot feel existent in the mind of the other. Such patients, often labeled borderline, may require emotionally available therapists or analysts willing to extend themselves beyond the traditional confines of analytic therapy (cf. Bacal, 1985, on optimal responsiveness). A colleague has told me of a patient who asked to have her therapist telephone her at a specified time each day. After several months, this became unnecessary, as the patient became more able to feel her continued existence both in the mind of her therapist and gradually in her own experience. Another gave her therapist books to take with him on vacation to make sure that he would remember her when he was gone. A third patient gave me a refrigerator magnet that was also a Christmas decoration. Asked about the magnet in February, I said I was putting it away with my holiday things, and the patient became very dejected. It turned out that the purpose of the magnet from the patient's point of view was to remind me of the patient, thereby keeping her in existence. Severely abused and tortured in childhood, this woman suffered severe discontinuities in her self-experience. She needed to use my memory of her from day to day in order to feel that she continued to exist as a member of the human species. A milder and more

common example of a patient's belief that he or she does not exist
for the therapist includes the patient's surprise that the analyst
remembers details emotionally significant to the patient. Such
memory opposes the patient's sense that out of sight is out of mind
and out of existence.

Another patient, when in extreme anxiety states, often called
friends and acquaintances just to see if they remembered him and
could tell him his name. Once they did, he was temporarily
reassured of his continuing existence. For several years he never
called his analyst when in these states, on the assumption, which
emerged later, that he would not be remembered, recognized, or
known. Meanwhile, he remained in an unsatisfying relationship
with a girlfriend, and the treatment seemed stalemated. Gradually
he came to feel safe enough to call his analyst for the type of
reassurance he had sought from friends. Together the patient and
therapist came to understand that prior to calling the therapist he
had felt that he did not exist for her. Now, with a sense of his
existence for the therapist, he could exist apart from the girlfriend
and live alone comfortably.

These examples illustrate difficulties people may have in
feeling the self as continuing in existence without the presence or
reassurance of another person. The problem, surely grounded in
early experiences of physical or emotional abandonment, is an
intersubjectively generated lack of the ability to use a particular
kind of selfobject experience, perhaps a selfobject experience as
fundamental as Kohut's mirroring and idealizing. Providing this
selfobject experience might be described as holding in memory,
and the patient's use of it as feeling existent for the other. In
extreme forms, deficits in this capacity may cause a person to feel
lost, as if she or he is disappearing, or even completely nonexistent,
when there is no immediate perception of her or his existence or
significance for another person. In the intersubjective context of
treatment, such patients may feel extremely needy, demanding, or
baffling to their therapists. We may respond by falling back on our
familiar defenses—distancing by diagnosis, for example.

There are various ways in which we can work with the impasses
that then occur, depending on both the patient's and our own
particular patterns of experiencing, or organizing principles.
Other variables include the history of the particular bond estab-

lished in treatment and the therapist's degree of comfort with a range of interventions and responses. Sometimes the consistent presence and responsiveness of the therapist who has become aware of the nature of the difficulty is enough. The treatment of the man who called people to hear them say his name was helped in this way. Often all or most of the process must go on silently, though articulation sometimes helps. If I try to articulate the difficulty but nothing changes, I know I must be content to work in the nonverbal realm.

Sometimes, telephone calls or keeping Christmas magnets up all year may be necessary. Such interventions probably deserve the name of transitional phenomena, though perhaps in the opposite sense of that originally intended by Winnicott (1958). A more traditional intervention based on Winnicott's idea of transitional phenomena would be for the analyst to lend patient a small item from her office to keep while the analyst is on vacation. The reverse is illustrated by the patient who gave her analyst books to take with him on vacation. During his first vacation, she had slashed her-self—not as a suicide attempt but as an effort to feel her own reality. Once she found a way to assure herself that he would remember her, she had no more major difficulties with his vacations.

A particularly evocative response by a therapist aware of a patient's severe difficulty with feeling held in memory and existent for the other is the following: The patient, who had extreme difficulty with both object constancy in the more traditional sense and with feeling continuously existent for herself and for the other, deteriorated each year as her analyst's long vacation approached. One year the analyst, who always wore a set of three bracelets, lent the patient one to wear while she was gone. Not only did the patient have something that belonged to the therapist to use as a transi-tional object, but the patient also knew that her therapist would frequently be aware of the missing third bracelet and would thus remember the patient—hold her in existence—during the vacation. Parenthetically, we may note that the meaning of gifts or loans, to or from analysts, may often lie in the transitional realm and may sometimes, like other transitional phenomena, be spoiled by too much analysis. In other situations, discussion may allow both participants in the analytic field to understand the meaning of the gift and in that way further the analysis.

Interventions in which an analyst takes some action to help the patient feel held in memory may seem unnecessary to analysts who believe that verbal interpretation makes up the entire realm of psychoanalytic work. We can respond to this objection in two ways. First, the trend in psychoanalysis for many years has been to expand the range of patients with whom we can work and to understand human beings as motivated primarily by relational concerns. Increasingly we are working with people whose difficulties seem to originate in preverbal interactions or lack of interactions with early caretakers. Often we find that purely verbal responses to these difficulties leave the patient feeling lost, misunderstood, or despairing. Relying solely on verbal responses may result in the impasses and treatment failures we experience from time to time.*

A second, and more important, response to those who hold that the psychoanalytic endeavor is purely verbal is my belief that our difficulties in noticing deficits in feeling held in memory, and our discomfort with interventions that could establish or restore this experience, may be based on the mistaken notion that the healthy person is self-sufficient. I believe, on the contrary, that human beings are interdependent by nature. The sense of self as cohesive, continuous, and positively valued develops and continues in an intersubjective context. I often find it necessary to remind myself and my patients that needing others is nothing to be ashamed of. In his posthumously published *How Does Analysis Cure?* Kohut (1984) eloquently challenged the separation–individuation conception of maturity:

> Self psychology holds that self-selfobject relationships form the essence of psychological life from birth to death, that a move from dependency (symbiosis) to independence (autonomy) in the psychological sphere is no more possible, let alone desirable, than a corresponding move from a life dependent on oxygen to a life independent of it in the biological sphere. The developments that

---

*Of course no response or intervention will be helpful unless the therapist is comfortable working in that way—although it may be on the outer edge of her or his comfort zone. The response must also come from some understanding of the nature the patient's particular suffering, whether or not the patient can articulate this. In addition, no single intervention can be recommended; what is necessary, instead, is to recognize the patient's efforts to create a reliable bond.

characterize normal psychological life must, in our view, be seen in the changing nature of the relationship between the self and its selfobjects, but not in the self's relinquishment of selfobjects. (p. 47)

If we accept Kohut's view of our lifelong need for others and begin to recognize the centrality of the need to feel existent for the other, we can understand some clinical and everyday phenomena. One therapist, for example, had two surgeries several years apart. He found overall that after the first operation, when he called patients from the hospital as soon as he could, his patients reported much less distress than after the second operation, when he did not call his patients as quickly. Even generally high-functioning patients felt disoriented and lost as the days went by and they heard nothing. They knew that no news was good news. The therapist's death would have been reported to them. The experience was not exactly of the loss of the therapist. Instead patients lost the sense that they continued to exist in the therapist's memory, their familiar sense of the relationship within which they were coming to possess a sense of their own existence.

Similar phenomena can be found in everyday life. Anyone who has moved a long distance will have had the experience of being able to maintain some friendships but not others over time and distance. I once had a friend—a close friend, I thought—in Seattle who told me that when I moved to New York, it would be the end of our friendship. She would feel that I no longer really existed and that she would no longer exist for me. No measures I took to convince her otherwise were successful in overcoming these convictions. We might speculate that to maintain a friendship over time and distance, both friends need to have achieved both object constancy and the sense of being held in memory by the other.

To return to the clinical situation, I am suggesting that many misunderstandings and impasses result both from patient difficulties feeling held in memory, and therefore in existence, and from analysts' reluctance, or inability, to be emotionally available enough to struggle with the patient toward an understanding of this problem. The sense of existence comes from the reliable experience of existence for the other, of being known, remembered, and understood. Some stalemates can be overcome if we recognize, welcome, and support the efforts of patients to create transitional means of reassuring themselves of their continuing existence and importance for us until this ability is firmly established. The pragmatist shift to an epistemology of meaning, and to an ontology of perspectival realism, gives us great flexibility in understanding these clinical phenomena. Our clinical theories must support and articulate such relational understanding.

Misunderstanding often seems to be the normal state of the psychoanalytic triad—the two subjectivities and the intersubjective field that includes them. If some fundamental emotional safety exists, however, analyst and patient together can attain understanding by continually working through, in a fallibilistic spirit, the small and large misunderstandings.

CHAPTER 11

How Does Psychoanalytic Understanding Heal?*

> To cure rarely, to relieve suffering often, and
> to comfort always.
>
> —Old medical injunction

As I neared the completion of this book, a patient announced to me one day, "I don't think I care about being understood. I don't expect people to understand me. I want to feel loved and cared for whether I am understood or not." He thought that just such a feeling of being loved and cared for was what was working in his treatment. This patient thus forces me to articulate the implications of my pragmatic and intersubjective view of understanding for a theory of therapeutic action or efficacy. An honest pragmatist must, of course, acknowledge in a fallibilistic spirit that our clinical theories are never more than working hypotheses. We must also, like the ancient physicians, admit that genuine cure is a comparatively rare occurrence.

Nevertheless, the "cash value" (James, 1907) of any psychoanalytic theory lies in its account of cure. I have placed the idea of understanding in the center of the epistemology and clinical theory of psychoanalysis. Now I must explain the implications of this position for the question of therapeutic action, a question that

*Dr. Peter Lessem and I collaborated in writing early versions of some sections of this chapter.

has a long and thoughtful history. This history reflects a gradual shift from the interpretation-and-insight view toward an explicit emphasis on the healing power of relational and emotional understanding.

THE EFFICACY OF PSYCHOANALYSIS

Since Breuer and Freud's (1895) *Studies on Hysteria,* it has been clear that psychoanalytic treatment in the hands of a skilled practitioner can be helpful. On the other hand, why this should be so and how the process works have never been clear for very long to very many people. As both participants in and observers of the psychoanalytic process, we often find ourselves at a loss to articulate the reasons for successes and failures. The question of therapeutic efficacy has, however, obvious practical significance. If we know what helps, we will do it, unless the cost proves too great to us as therapists. More than any other, perhaps, this question bridges the gap between psychoanalytic theory and practice, and it relies on the hermeneutic pragmatism that characterizes my account of psychoanalytic understanding. The question of therapeutic efficacy, precisely because it is so difficult to resolve, spans the history of psychoanalysis.

Breuer and Freud (1895) originally thought that people recover from "hysterias" by recalling early traumas and by the cathartic reexperience of the emotional states associated with these early traumas, that is, by abreaction. Once Freud adopted his topographical view of the mind, he asserted that analysis cures by making the unconscious conscious. Wishful conflicts, once acknowledged, lose their power, and symptoms disappear. With the coming of Freud's structural theory, this process meant that ego control replaces id wishes and that mature organization supplants infantile chaos. With little change, this drive-based understanding of psychoanalytic cure persists today in Freudian ego psychology and Kleinian analysis.

Starting in the 1930s, however, dissenting voices emerged. In Budapest, Ferenczi, who stressed the emotional quality of the unique psychoanalytic bond (Bacal & Newman, 1990), wondered whether the relationship itself might not be the curative factor. In addition, he emphasized the therapeutic potential of regression and emotional reliving in the transference. Viewing the traditional reserved analytic attitude as inappropriate to heal the "traumatized child" in the patient, he thought analysts needed to be more responsive. They ought to make the analytic relationship a place of safety in which the patient could relive the original trauma in a context that is different from the original one, thereby making it possible for the patient to experience a new beginning.

Ferenczi underscored the analyst's contribution to the therapeutic bond. He stressed (1) the ways in which what the analyst provides to the patient differs from what the patient has experienced in the past, (2) the analyst's love for the patient, and (3) the importance of reducing impediments in the analyst to understanding and connecting emotionally with the patient. The first two of these concerns figured prominently in Ferenczi's remarkably up-to-date discussions on the treatment of trauma. For example, Ferenczi (1988) contrasted his view with Freud's:

An abreaction of quantities of the trauma is not enough. The situation must be different from the actually traumatic one in order to make possible a different, favorable outcome. (p. 108)

If the present process is to have a different outcome from the original trauma, then the victim of traumatogenic shock must be offered something in reality, at least as much caring attention, or a genuine intention to provide it, as a traumatized child must have. (p. 28)

No analysis can succeed if we do not succeed in really loving the patient. Every patient has the right to be regarded and cared for as an ill-treated, unhappy child. (p. 130)

Without discounting the power of transference, Ferenczi underscored the actual personality of the analyst in the therapeutic situation. Believing that the analyst's personality strongly influences the course of treatment, he criticized the overvaluation of theoretical insight. Personal qualities of the analyst, as well as feelings of liking, interest in, or indifference toward patients, come through and evoke unconscious responses from the patient (p. 191). Ferenczi was a solitary voice stressing the profoundly relational nature of the psychoanalytic process, including the need for attention to countertransference. This attention, he believed, facilitates the analyst's understanding of and emotional availability to the patient. Toward these ends, Ferenczi experimented with the radical innovation of mutual analysis. He hoped that by allowing patients to hear and explore his responses and transferences to them he would reduce the interference of his countertransference and what he called his "obtuseness."

In Britain, Strachey (1934), in his remarkable paper "The Nature of the Therapeutic Action of Psycho-Analysis," described the curative role of the therapeutic relationship. Within the safety of the analytic bond, the patient could more easily make use of interpretations. Strachey described the elements that contribute to the patient's ability to integrate interpretations. These include the patient's will to recover and capacity to assimilate reasonable arguments, as well as the relationship with the therapist. Strachey believed that the patient's positive attachment to the analyst in the transference makes therapeutic change possible through modification of the superego. The patient assimilates the analyst into his or her tripartite psychic structure as an auxiliary superego. This auxiliary superego, a good object, differs from the bad objects of the patient's past. Effective, or "mutative," interpretations help the patient become aware of the contrast between the archaic fantasy object and the real analytic object. The resulting introjection of this less aggressive, more benign object into the patient's superego modifies superego aggression, thereby creating interference with the habitual neurotic process. For Strachey, psychic change results from the internalization of the analyst as a good object via mutative interpretation.

Also in Britain, several analysts with a radically social conception of human nature challenged drive theory. They suggested that the basic human striving is for connection with others, often, in deference to Freud, called "objects."* This major transformation of theory—perhaps even a paradigm shift—to a relational model is still in progress. Greenberg and Mitchell (1983), as well as Bacal

*Freud's conception of the object probably came from philosopher Franz Brentano, from whom he took five courses. Brentano held that intentionality, or reference to an object, defines psychic life. Thus, to think is to think something, to desire is to want something, and so on.

and Newman (1990), have extensively explored this change in theoretical focus.

Ian Suttie (1935), for example, who I suspect has been neglected because he was so straightforwardly radical, understood human beings as motivated primarily by the need and desire for companionship and love. He saw hatred as frustration in the search for love. Differentiating sexuality from tenderness, he accused the Freudians of reductionistic pansexualism. Suttie complained, in addition, of what he called the taboo on tenderness, or antiemotionalism, in scientific psychology, in society, and particularly among psychoanalysts. He thought that society underappreciates and undercompensates the work of mothers and nurses, and he attributed this phenomenon to a general aversion to tenderness. Noting that society views as unmanly tenderness for people or animals, he thought that men had often substituted sexuality for the love and tenderness that were taboo for them. In Suttie's view, Freud, by building the taboo on tenderness into his theory, reduced tenderness, love, and companionship to derivatives of sexuality.

Suttie believed that psychoanalysis provides an opportunity to restore lost or damaged capacities to find companionship and love. He liked to quote Ferenczi's saying, "It is the physician's love that heals the patient," and he felt that this position has enormous practical bearing:

> If we do not like a patient we are hopelessly handicapped in treating him. No amount of technical skill, theoretical knowledge or conscientiousness will atone for the absence of a sympathetic understanding and the capacity to "put oneself in the patient's place." (p. 74)

Suttie believed that all mental illness, no matter what its biological concomitants or how isolative it appears, is a disturbance in social relatedness. He therefore provided a developmental, and in today's terminology, thoroughly intersubjective, account of the development of symptoms:

> Mind is so intimately and constantly dependent upon interplay with other minds that any disturbance of its *interpsychic* [Suttie's word]

relationships *further* alters the affected mind in a "vicious circle." The loss of touch with others produces a vast number of secondary symptoms, reparative, compensatory, defensive, defiant, etc., and produces *in the observer's mind* the illusion that the patient's trouble is of relatively recent, definite and sudden onset, whereas in reality much of the disturbance and distress is due to emotions evoked by the impairment of companionship (of love and of interest) in the distant past. Further, every lapse from sociability on the part of the patient produces an *antipathetic response from his social environment*, which in turn has its repercussions upon himself. Thus a vicious circle of protest and counter-protest and misunderstanding is set up. In consequence the patient is alienated not so much of his own accord as by a sort of *emotional ostracism* on the part of others. He did not intend to become isolated, even unconsciously. He was forced into it. (p. 182)

This intersubjective account of psychopathology has important implications for understanding the therapeutic action of psychoanalysis. For Suttie the task of psychotherapy is "to induce the patient to lay aside her age-old defenses against the infantile dread of isolation, and to find an adequate substitute in adult love and interest-companionship" (p. 203). In another place, he claimed that psychotherapy involves "the *overcoming of the barriers to loving and feeling oneself loved*, and not the removal of fear-imposed inhibitions to the expression of innate, anti-social, egoistic, and sensual desires" (pp. 53–54).

Like Suttie, Fairbairn challenged the fundamental conceptual structure of Freudian psychoanalysis when he claimed that human beings are object-seeking from birth. He sought to replace the Freudian emphasis on impulse and drive with a focus on how people maintain crucial ties in the face of neglect or frustration of vital relational needs. According to Fairbairn, a person copes with the frustration that results from unsatisfactory early object relationships by splitting psychic experience. The unification of the split ego, or split psyche, became for Fairbairn the aim of psychoanalytic therapy. He regarded the split ego as an internal "closed system" that evolved as a reaction to the effects of unsatisfactory early object relationships. Thus, Fairbairn (1952) believed that "the chief aim of psycho-analytical treatment is to promote a maximum synthesis of the structure into which the original ego has been split"

(p. 380). To do so, the patient needs help to release bad objects from repression and to dissolve "libidinal" ties to them in order to become free to form healthier object relationships. As Bacal (1990) paraphrases Fairbairn, "Interpretation alone is insufficient; the patient's maintaining his inner world as a closed system has been partially determined *by his sense of hopelessness in obtaining any satisfaction from objects in external reality upon whom he might allow himself to become dependent*" (p. 357).

To feel safe enough to risk releasing internalized bad objects from repression (i.e., to experience them as bad), and to experience them in the transference, the patient must experience the analyst as a good object (Bacal & Newman, 1990, p. 152). In Fairbairn's words, "It is the actual relationship between the patient and the analyst [that] constitutes the decisive factor in psychoanalytical, no less than in any other form of psychotherapeutic care" (p. 385). More precisely, "the relationship between the patient and the analyst is not just the relationship involved in the transference, but the total relationship existing between the patient and the analyst as persons" (p. 379). This tie with " a reliable and beneficent parental figure" (p. 377) was the relationship denied to the patient in childhood.

The most influential contributor to the paradigm shift to a relational model is Winnicott (1958, 1965). Focusing on the similarities between the mother–infant relationship and the analytic situation, he saw analysts as providing a holding environment similar to that furnished by good-enough mothering. A regressive experience in such an analysis, he thought, frees the patient from the persistent dominance of a compliant false-self organization, thereby making possible the emergence of a spontaneous, true self. Winnicott's work on play and on transitional experience opened our eyes to the wide range of human experience, especially including the creative regions, that has relational meaning. He thus helped us to see nonverbal and playful activities of bonding both in childhood and adulthood. His highlighting of "primary maternal preoccupation" in infancy, with its considerable demands on the mother, parallels his emphasis on the management of the limits of analysts' emotional availability. He said, more than half seriously, that his patients had to "queue up" for their regressions (Little, 1990). Similarly, Gotthold (1992) notes both the necessity and difficulties of analytic wholeheartedness with patients like those about whom Winnicott wrote.

Bowlby, who has been ignored in British psychoanalysis both because of his ethological analogies and because his thought was radical, articulated the bonding hypothesis even more clearly than Winnicott did. In his last book, Bowlby (1988) summarized his life's work under two headings: (1) the importance for psychoanalysis of considering how the actual conditions of a child's emotional environment affect the person's development and (2) the developmental primacy of experiences of attachment, separation, and loss, or, as he sometimes said, the making and breaking of emotional bonds.

Although Bowlby rejected drive theory and the Kleinian language of Winnicott, he saw the clinical work of Winnicott as most closely allied with his own thinking. However, while Bowlby saw the task of therapy as clearly focused on issues of relatedness, he viewed the process itself as insight-oriented. Bowlby acknowledged his similarity to Kohut on this issue. What is remarkable is how clearly Bowlby (1988) articulated the basic condition for the possibility of any healing through insight:

> The first [task] is to provide the patient with a secure base from which he can explore the various unhappy and painful aspects of his life, past and present, many of which he finds it difficult or perhaps impossible to think about and reconsider without a trusted companion to provide support, encouragement, sympathy, and, on occasion, guidance. (p. 138)

Other aspects of psychoanalysis emphasized by Bowlby were exploration, comparison of divergent experiences and perspectives, and understanding. But the creation of emotional security was Bowlby's lifelong interest. He compared the secure-base-providing role of the therapist with "that of a mother who provides her child with a secure base from which to explore the world" (p. 140). The therapist provides a zone of safety in which the patient can explore the effects of his or her personal history—of trauma, neglect, or other trouble—on self-experience in the past and present.

Michael Balint, an analysand of Ferenczi, imported Ferenczi's ideas into the group of British psychoanalysts who embraced the social conception of human beings. Balint made important additions to Ferenczi's thinking about the importance of the patient–analyst relationship. Balint viewed psychoanalysis as a two-person or two-body psychology, not the one-person psychology of traditional analytic therapy. Like his mentor Ferenczi, therefore, he encouraged careful attention to the analyst's contribution to the therapeutic situation. Moreover, in Balint's words, "The events during an analysis are not determined by the patient's associations and transference, or by the analyst's interpretation, but by an interaction between the two" (Balint, 1953, as quoted in Bacal & Newman, 1990, p. 127). The course of an analysis, Balint maintained, is not a simple product of the analysand's early experience. It also results from the current relations among the patient, the analyst, and the ethos of the analytic situation.*

Balint's relational theory of the genesis of psychopathology, especially his conception of "the basic fault," engendered his view of therapeutic action. His "basic fault" referred to a major discrepancy, or gap, between a patient's needs in infancy and the capacity of the people in the child's early environment to respond to these needs. By regressing in the transference to the level of the basic fault, the patient attempts to form the needed reparative relationship with the analyst. Once regressed to this level, the patient can discover that rigidly maintained, self-protective conditions for relating and loving are no longer necessary. In the phase Balint (1968) called "the new beginning" (pp. 131–132), a person can relinquish these rigid conditions.

Meanwhile, the American Hans Loewald (1960a), working in ego psychology with its objectivist assumptions but influenced by the pioneering British psychoanalysts, wrote an extraordinary paper, "On the Therapeutic Action of Psychoanalysis." Loewald argued that the relational features of the analyst's interpretive activity are central to the therapeutic action of psychoanalysis. In his words, the "resumption of ego development is contingent on the relationship with the new object, the analyst" (p. 221). "The newness consists in the patient's rediscovery of the early paths of the development of object relations leading to a new way of relating to objects and of being oneself" (p. 229). This new relational

---

*This idea resembles my intersubjective conception of the psychoanalytic triad (Chapter 2).

experience for the patient comes about largely through the analyst's interpretation of the patient's transference distortion. "The chiselling away of transference distortions" (p. 225) permits the process of identification that Loewald, like Strachey, saw as central to the new object tie. Growth occurs, Loewald believed, by the internalization of relational exchanges between the self and the other. The analyst provides regulating and organizing functions for the patient by interpretation in a way analogous to the mother's care for the child. For Loewald, the patient internalizes the interaction process in which the analyst's interpretations supply an "integrative experience" for the patient. This process mediates between the patient's idiosyncratic, childish beliefs and the analyst's more highly differentiated organization.

To summarize, we could say that each of these authors—Ferenczi, Strachey, Suttie, Fairbairn, Winnicott, Bowlby, Balint, and Loewald—conceived of psychoanalysis as a return to the road not taken by the patient because it was not available to her or him as a child. These theoreticians believed that the lack of crucial attachment bonds, or primary emotional ties, prevents the emergence of a robust self. In analysis the patient returns to the conditions of infancy, not in a regressive sense but as an emotional opportunity for a much needed attachment that makes possible progressive development in adulthood.

Because of Strachey and Loewald, the question of how analysis works has been prominent in recent psychoanalytic thought. We turn now to how this issue has been approached within self psychology, both by Kohut and by some of those who have continued to develop self psychological theory. In the spirit of inquiry and growth of theory proposed by Kohut (1977, p. 312), I have slightly modified Kohut's (1984) question "How does analysis cure?" to ask: How does psychoanalytic understanding heal?

Kohut's (1977) explicit answer was that optimal frustration promotes transmuting internalization. By "frustration" he seems to have meant the disruptions and misunderstanding that inevitably occur, even in a treatment characterized by the empathic inquiry and empathically informed interpretations by the analyst. If adequately analyzed, these disruptions of the self–selfobject milieu enable the patient to internalize the analyst's selfobject functions—mirroring and soothing, for example. The patient thus builds up newly cohesive, stable, and positively valued psychic structure, or selfhood.

Kohut reaffirmed this view of cure in his 1984 book, emphasizing that frustration is inherent in the analytic process, which can provide only understanding and explanation, not gratification of the needs being understood. In his words, "It is the accretion of psychic structure via an optimal frustration of the analysand's needs or wishes that is provided for the analysand in the form of correct interpretations that constitutes the essence of the cure" (p. 108). Yet in this same work, Kohut also hinted that while self psychologically oriented analysis makes no major technical departures from classical analysis, something besides interpretation may be involved in psychoanalytic cure. In his account of the disruptions that lead to transmuting internalization of psychic structure, Kohut emphasized the mending or repair of the self–selfobject tie, or empathic bond, between analyst and patient (Jaenicke, 1987). Although, to my knowledge, Kohut never said that the process of mending a broken tie in the present makes possible a partial healing of the self broken in the past—his explicit emphasis was more on structure-building than on healing—his work suggests that self psychologically informed psychoanalysis works in this way. In addition, when this occurs, it may give the patient a feeling of hope that further healing is possible.

In this vein, Kohut (1981) suggested that, much as he wished to regard empathic understanding simply as a scientific tool for gathering data, he had been forced to recognize and admit that empathy itself might be curative. Thus part of Kohut's legacy to psychoanalysis is the recognition that both relatedness and empathy-informed interpretation are crucial to psychoanalytic cure. The open questions concern the relative importance of these two elements and the nature of the relationship between them.

In fact Kohut placed the formation of self-consolidating emotional connections squarely in the foreground of analytic thought and practice. The selfobject conception, self psychology's theoretical heart, placed the ability of emotional bonds to strengthen self-experience right in the center of emotional experience, development, and cure. In other words, Kohut too thought that analysis gives patients a second chance at healthy emotional development based on attachment. Nevertheless, this emphasis surfaced most clearly in his later works.

As noted above, Kohut (1977) originally claimed that change occurs through transmuting internalization. In his view the patient takes in forms of self-experience made newly available by selfobject experience in treatment, especially while mending nontraumatically disrupted selfobject bonds. Gradually the patient incorporates forms of self-experience—ideals, ambitions, enthusiasms, firmness, for example—from his or her therapist's reasonably consistent responsiveness, presumably missing in the patient's childhood. Kohut accounted for the increased experience of self-cohesiveness, self-continuity, and positive self-experience by these "transmuting internalizations."

While internalization is undoubtedly a spatial metaphor that is vulnerable to criticism as overly concrete and simple, the transmuting part of the inferred process is more abstract and complex. The patient inevitably and continually transforms the current selfobject experience with the analyst according to already organized preconceptions inferred from her or his emotional history—importantly including the history of experience with the analyst—and thus gains new psychological organization or structure. In addition, it is clear that Kohut meant that selfobject experience changes the patient over time into a stronger person with a firmer and more positive sense of self. In his last writings Kohut (1977, 1984) placed more emphasis on this kind of change. However, he was reluctant to do this because he wanted empathy to be understood as a method of investigation, not as a direct route to cure through being kind. His own accumulated experience, however, led him to acknowledge that something *was* curative about the experience of feeling understood (1981).

An intersubjective account of psychoanalytic understanding places the process of organizing and reorganizing experience at its center (Stolorow et al., 1987; Stolorow & Atwood, 1992). Stolorow (1994) has moved away from a transformational view that sees organizing principles as replaced or radically modified in treatment. He believes instead that we acquire an expanded repertoire of principles for organizing experience more flexibly. Relational predicaments that closely resemble the intersubjective situations in which we formed our original assumptions can evoke them again. Yet we know that people do become more flexible, more moderate, more generous, and more content. How does this happen?

ATTACHMENT, SELFOBJECT EXPERIENCE, AND THERAPEUTIC EFFICACY

Psychoanalytic understanding is, among other things, a form of loving, and it can be experienced in that way by the patient. It differs from empathy, which is value-neutral and can be used to hurt people. Psychoanalytic understanding, as it characterizes both practitioner and process, is unequivocally propatient (Tolpin, 1991). Although patients may not recognize for a long time that we are on their side, we must know that we are. If we cannot find or maintain this attitude with a given patient, we ought to consult our colleagues and, if necessary, refer the patient. Often we can recognize our inability to stay on the side of a patient in the kind of humor—is it ironic or sarcastic?—we use in speaking with colleagues about this patient. Another clue comes in our use of diagnostic labels like "borderline" or "hysteric," which denigrate the patient and short-circuit the interplay of psychoanalytic understanding. Labeling may have other functions, of course, but none of these, in my view, furthers the process of understanding.

Being propatient, although only one part of cure or healing, is, like emotional availability, a necessary condition for its possibility. It probably forms part of that emotional availability so crucial to the attachment process that I see as the core of the therapeutic efficacy of psychoanalytic treatment.

What then is the connection between attachment and emotional healing? Clearly not all psychological change requires a crucial emotional bond to an analyst or therapist. Drugs, cognitive-behavioral therapies, and strategic or systemic family therapies operate—or claim to—without such bonds. I believe that an adequate psychoanalytic conception of therapeutic action through understanding requires that we look again at the selfobject conception.

The cornerstone of self psychological theory is the idea of selfobject experience. In my view the particular human being who provides selfobject experience matters profoundly. Thus, we can clarify the selfobject notion by reference to ideas that have emerged from research into early attachments. Prominent attachment theorists include Bowlby, Ainsworth, Sroufe, and Main. In contrast to classical psychoanalytic theory, attachment theory asserts that needs for safety and security, rather than for reduction of physiological drive tensions, lead to the formation of a bond between caretaker and infant (Bowlby, 1979).

Self psychologists and attachment researchers share in common a central belief in the overriding importance of the tendency of human beings to form strong emotional bonds to individual others. Both believe that this tendency to form strong bonds with special others is at the core of human functioning and human psychology throughout life. As Bacal and Newman (1990) point out, both approaches stress the importance for healthy development of relationships with phase-appropriately responsive and supportive figures. Additionally, both theoretical traditions maintain that this tendency is present in the infant and continues throughout adult life till death. Further, both believe that a principal feature of competent personality functioning and mental health is the ability to form emotional ties with people, in both the careseeking and caretaking roles.

Significant differences, nevertheless, exist between the two theories. Self psychologists view self-development as originating in, and maintained by, the experience of support from responsive and idealizable others. Self psychology calls these experiences "selfobject" to suggest that we feel people who provide them as supports to our selfhood, not primarily as subjects of their own experience. When caretakers disappear or fail, the child can often use another available adult to supply the needed ideals, validation, and support.

Attachment theorists, partly to the contrary, see the development of a self as contingent on reliable emotional bonds to particular caretakers. Recent infant research views infants as originally capable of and disposed to such ties. The stability of these bonds provides a sense of safety for the child, a secure base (Bowlby, 1988) from which the child can venture forth to explore the world. To lose such an irreplaceable caretaker can be profoundly traumatizing, and the loss may never entirely heal.

Attachment theory has been conceptualized by its researchers in behavioral, dyadic terms. Generally, theorists and scientists in the attachment tradition—Bowlby, Ainsworth, Sroufe, and many others—have emphasized the behaviorally observable effects of the formation and disruption of attachment. They also correlate security of attachment with various abilities and behaviors later in childhood and adolescence. Conceived in measurable and behavioral terms, attachment theory has become a prominent paradigm in infant research.

Yet attachment theorists sometimes neglect the subjective experience of attachment, including the personal meanings of attachment, separation, and loss. According to Greenberg and Mitchell (1983), Bowlby does not "account for the emotional need for and meaning of attachment and relationship in the development of a distinctly human self" (p. 187).

Self psychology, on the contrary, addresses the *experience* of attachment and loss. An example of this is the recent interest among self psychologists in the importance of the significant other for the patterning of self-experience. This is evident in Stolorow et al.'s (1987) intersubjectivity theory, Bacal's (1990) and Bacal and Newman's (1990) work delineating the object relational "bridges" to self psychology, Beebe and Lachmann's (1988) emphasis on mutual influence structures in their work on the development of representations, Fosshage's (1992b, 1994) work on the organizational conception of transference and the self in the relational matrix, and Lessem's (1992) work on the relational patterning of affective experience. Self psychology now addresses many of the same issues that have occupied attachment researchers.

To account for certain clinical phenomena—especially of loss, idiosyncratic personality development, the repetition of painful relational experience, and the uniqueness of each psychoanalytic treatment—self psychology needs to include attachment within its central theoretical ideas. According to the attachment theorists, however, attachment is always to a particular individual. In the words of Bacal and Newman (1990), self psychological theory "does not provide for an acknowledgment of the importance of object specificity" (p. 231). "In focusing on the experience of selfobject *function*, . . . self-psychology theory has lost sight of the object that provides that function" (p. 230). If self psychology is to fulfill its promise, it must find a way to take the particularity of relational experience into theoretical account. I believe that *stable attachments form a necessary condition for the possibility of "primary selfobject relatedness" (a term explained below). Such relatedness in turn is indispensable to the integration of affect that is crucial to cohesive, continuous, and positively colored self-experience.*

Let me add a point of clarification: My focus here is not the question of the link between self psychology and object relations theories. For my purpose there is no need to decide whether self psychology is truly part of object relations theory or whether object relations theories in some interesting ways anticipated self psychology. Others deeply versed in both ways of thinking (Brandchaft, 1986; Bacal & Newman, 1990; P. Ornstein, 1991) have extensively considered these questions.

Instead we must use the empirical findings of attachment research to clarify and enrich what self psychology—a psychoanalytic theory that relies on introspection and empathy as its methods of collecting data—has taught us about the relational origins of self-experience. In "Introspection, Empathy, and Psychoanalysis: An Examination of the Relationship Between Mode of Observation and Theory," Kohut (1959) articulated the difference between empirical theories and those based primarily on the data gained by introspection and empathy. In his words:

> Some concepts used by psychoanalysis are not abstractions founded on introspective observation or empathic introspection, but are derived from data obtained through other methods of observation. Such concepts must be compared with the theoretical abstractions based on psychoanalytic observations; they are not, however, identical with them. (p. 221)

Attachment theories "are derived from data obtained through other methods of observation." I do not, therefore, propose a simple merger of attachment theory with self psychology. These theories belong to different realms of discourse, to distinct conceptual schemes. Nevertheless, awareness of the findings of attachment research will expand the range of our empathy and will help us refine and clarify some theoretical notions of self psychology. Genuinely psychoanalytic theories always include "introspection and empathy *as an essential constituent*" (Kohut, 1959, p. 209). Still, those who seek to develop psychoanalytic theories must consider empirical findings and use these to improve our powers of empathic observation. Let us therefore examine the connections among selfobject experience, attachment, understanding, and psychoanalytic cure.

Primary and Derivative Selfobject Relatedness

In its brief history, self psychology has variously conceived the selfobject as person, function, dimension of experience, and vitalizing experience. Here I present my own developing view of the selfobject experience in secure attachments.

I will begin by distinguishing the selfobject connection from other forms of experienced relatedness. First, it differs from the I–Thou, or subject–subject, reciprocal connection, which defines a special kind of intersubjective field in which two people, either momentarily or fundamentally, stand in relation, at times perhaps mutually acknowledged, as subjects of experience. (Selfobject connection may, however, exist within this intersubjective form.) While prolonged I–Thou relatedness often sustains mutual selfobject relatedness, only when we describe the other felt as support for the self are we speaking of selfobject relatedness. Selfobject relatedness is an asymmetrical relational experience.[*] It can, however, exist for both people in a mutual relation of I and Thou. Aron (1992) says that the psychoanalytic relationship is at once mutual and asymmetrical. Similarly, we can view selfobject relatedness (asymmetrical by definition) as existing within an intersubjective field in which both people fully participate.

Second, selfobject relatedness differs from personal relatedness in the legal or philosophical sense (Macmurray, 1957). In these views, the person or self is an agent in relation to other agents. Likewise, selfobject relatedness is not interpersonal in the interactive sense understood by most Sullivanian psychoanalysts. Instead, selfobject relatedness is a thoroughly subjective relational experience.

[*] Lynn Preston (personal communication) believes that selfobject experience is intrinsically bidirectional, that both people must give and receive if selfobject experience is to occur.

Third, selfobject relatedness is not I–It, instrumental, or subject–object relatedness (in the philosophical, not the psychoanalytic, sense of an *object*), although things, including ideas and forms of culture, may sometimes serve secondary, or derivative, selfobject functions (a concept to be explained later in this chapter). The I–It relation is one of user to object or item. When we experience another as support for the stability of our self-experience, we do not automatically reduce the other to the status of a thing. The common reference to the "use" of another as selfobject may mislead us into thinking that the special personality of the other is irrelevant. We may drift into the assumption that the providers of selfobject experience are as interchangeable as similar objects of use. We cannot drive into any emotional gas station and order regular unleaded selfobject experience, as if anyone would do as well as anyone else. Kohut did not see people as replaceable items. He taught us, on the contrary, not to differentiate between archaic and mature selfobject needs as if the distinction were between I–It and I–Thou relatedness, between relatedness that is primarily self-gratifying and that which springs from a true desire to connect with others. Throughout life, mature people have many kinds of connections to other human beings and considerable flexibility in their relational capacities.

Selfobject relatedness is a special kind of relatedness that creates and maintains positive and stable self-experience. We may feel the other as a selfobject and simultaneously experience her or him as subject or as object. Selfobject experience can coexist with, and inhere in, various forms of relational experience. A person, for example, who normally treats me as an adversary may give me some grudging admiration that, at least temporarily, strengthens my self-respect. Essential to selfobject relatedness is its experiential character, its nature as subjective and as strengthening to a stable and positive sense of self. Self psychology uses the psychoanalytic access through introspection and empathy to discover selfobject relatedness. If introspection and empathy yield the only truly psychoanalytic knowledge, and if we can know selfobject relatedness only so, then selfobject relatedness is a fully psychoanalytic conception. (This inference displays the tight connection between Kohut's epistemological and methodological views [1959] and the central theoretical conceptions of self psychology.)

Expressions like "a form of relatedness," "a process of feeling

connection," and "experienced relatedness" are almost interchangeable. Two assumptions underlie this terminology. It implies,
first, that *experience*, whether self-experience or relational experience, *is process*. It is neither finished history nor encapsulated
moment. It always involves interplay or conversation, among past,
present, and future. Second, intentionally assuming that *relatedness
is process*, I prefer the word "relatedness" to the more static-sound-
ing "relation" or "relationship." This choice avoids making the
selfobject conception overly concrete. Instead, it retains experience-near and process-suggestive terms.

The intersubjectivity theory of Stolorow et al. (1987) provides
a theoretical framework for the specificity of the other and for the
particularity of selfobject relatedness. These authors insist repeatedly that an intersubjective field consists of the intersection and
interplay of two differently organized subjectivities. If, in such a
field, one subject finds the other a support for stable and positive
self-experience, it is that subject's experience of the particular other
as providing support that I designate "primary selfobject relatedness." This definition does not refer to infancy or maturity. It
requires only an important bond in which one or both subjects
experience the other as support for valued, cohesive selfhood.

Granted, not every intersubjective field is an attachment, or in
Bowlby's (1979) words, an "affectional bond." Still, selfobject
relatedness is the person's experience, at any age, of a significant
human other or attachment figure as support for the establishment, development, and maintenance of continuous, cohesive,
and positive self-experience.* I name this experience "primary
selfobject relatedness," and I believe that it inheres only in important emotional ties.

Undoubtedly, other self-vitalizing experiences can be important in childhood and adulthood. Many people feel, for example,
that some form of physical activity strengthens their sense of self.
Others gain a similar sense of self-vitalization from music or other
experiences of human culture or natural beauty. Let us call these

*The question of negative experience of a significant other arises here, either as "bad
selfobject" (an oxymoron, I think) or, as George Atwood (personal communication, 1994)
puts it, "people we may rely on negatively to support our sense of self, i.e., as counterex-
amples of who we are, where we solidify our sense of self through sharpening our contrast
with particular others." I do not claim that selfobject experience is the only psychologically
important experience we have of significant others, just that it is the only type that heals.

secondary forms of self-vitalization "derivative selfobject experience" (no reference to instinctual derivatives intended). This broader category of selfobject experiences is implicitly relational. The usefulness of these secondary selfobject experiences derives from primary selfobject relatedness in attachment bonds. Deprived of primary selfobject relatedness, people usually find that selfobject experience of these nonhuman forms only fleetingly sustains a sense of self. Self psychologists have observed that the ability to use this larger class of experience improves, expands, and becomes more flexible once the basic need for primary selfobject relatedness has found appropriate response in significant emotional bonds.

Selfobject experience, therefore, is a large class of both primary and derivative self-strengthening phenomena, within which selfobject relatedness is the primary and indispensable form. The derivative forms, implicitly and derivatively relational, resemble Winnicott's (1958) transitional experience. They have their importance as developmental achievements in their own right or as transitory substitutes, at any age, for the special human relatedness called selfobject relatedness.

Both self psychology and attachment theories point toward new ideas of development and maturity. Kohut used the expression "archaic" to describe forms of early relatedness that he thought persisted in narcissistically disordered personalities. He assumed, however, an undifferentiated matrix in which the infant experiences the caretaker only as part of the self. Recent research (Lichtenberg, 1983; Daniel Stern, 1985) has, however, convinced most self psychologists that infants can recognize their caretakers from the earliest days of life and that they are born with sophisticated relational capacities. Attachment theories, in addition, see emotional bonds as a lifelong need in primates, including humans. Few of us now share the assumptions about infancy on which Kohut's characterization of early selfobject relatedness as "archaic" rested. We need, therefore, to ask ourselves what we could mean, if anything, by speaking of mature selfobject relatedness.

This whole distinction, I believe, needs to be laid to rest. Selfobject relatedness is neither mature nor immature. Almost everyone is born with the capacity for such relatedness, but not nearly everyone is born into an emotional environment that makes this experience readily available in stable, secure attachments. Without such a human environment, we go about, as if starved for relational oxygen, seeking substitutes in anxious attachments, substances, or compulsive activity. Even these activities, however, are signs that a person has not given up. Relational maturation consists, not in relinquishing or diminishing the need for human attachments that can provide selfobject relatedness, not in realizing some ideal of independence from others, but in regaining and developing the original disposition to find well-being in the human world.

Immaturity, to repeat, is not attachment to significant others, nor is maturity a take-it-or-leave-it attitude toward selfobject relatedness. One of Kohut's most important contributions was a rejection of shame over our human need for relatedness. His conception of selfobject relatedness as self-constitutive affirmed the lifelong legitimacy of this need. If we water down the selfobject conception and make it overinclusive, we may then idealize a lesser need for human relatedness and intimacy. We then lose Kohut's fundamental insight into human nature, neglect the findings of attachment theories, and return to a version of maturity morality.

Primary selfobject relatedness is the person's experience, at any age, of a connection with a significant human other or attachment figure as support for the establishment, development, and maintenance of continuous, cohesive, positive self-experience. Such relatedness is crucial for learning to recognize, differentiate, and express a range of emotional experience. Primary selfobject relatedness, facilitated by optimal responsiveness (Bacal, 1985), provides a context in which we can comfortably come to include our own emotional life in an organized self. Then we no longer need to reject major portions of our self-experience, or to live a divided, disorganized, severely restricted life. Secure attachment makes primary selfobject relatedness possible. This emotional climate provides for the integration of affective experience into an organized and positively colored sense of self.

I believe psychoanalytic understanding creates in adulthood the opportunity for a second chance at such primary selfobject relatedness. There is no greater bonding agent than a prolonged attempt to make sense together of someone's emotional life.

CHAPTER 12

Illustration: Understanding Schreber

[God's] actions have been practiced against
me for years with the utmost cruelty and
disregard as only a beast deals with its prey.
            —DANIEL PAUL SCHREBER,
               Memoirs of My Nervous Illness

Such a father as this was by no means unsuitable
for transfiguration into a God in the affectionate
memory of [the] son from whom he had been so
early separated by death.
        —SIGMUND FREUD, "Psycho-Analytic Notes
              on an Autobiographical Account of a Case
                     of Paranoia (Dementia Paranoides)"

*R*ethinking Schreber, the German judge whose memoir Freud analyzed, illustrates many aspects of my view of understanding. The contrast between the reading of Schreber's memoir by Freud and those done from a self psychology–intersubjectivity theory point of view dramatically supports my contention that theory-choice matters, that it has practical clinical import. Simultaneously, it serves as an example of the need for fallibilism, or holding theory lightly, so we can notice and take account of new information or perspectives. In addition, my rethinking of Schreber demonstrates that we need not choose between self psychology and intersubjectivity theory, that concentrating on a patient's self-experience requires close attention to the intersubjective contexts of its past and present origins. The attempt to understand a person from writings alone has obvious and severe limits. Still, I believe this effort can illustrate my view that understanding comes from participation, from entry into the whole emotional predicament within which a person has organized and continues to organize experience, and from making sense together. I therefore complete my exploration of the nature of psychoanalytic understanding with a reexamination of the case Schreber made for himself.

Today we know Schreber because Freud wrote about him. Unlike Freud's own patients about whom he wrote, Schreber was never seen by Freud. This places Freud and a modern reader at the same starting point, except that we now have both Freud's (1911) "Psycho-Analytic Notes on an Autobiographical Account of a Case of Paranoia (Dementia Paranoides)" and considerable biographical research on Schreber, his family, and his psychiatrist Flechsig. No one has access to the vast array of nonverbal data on which the empathic–introspective method relies so heavily in clinical psychoanalysis (Schwaber, 1983). What we do have in common with Freud is a substantial autobiographical account of a psychosis, Schreber's *Denkwürdgikeiten eines Nervenkranken,* or *Memoirs of My Nervous Illness* (1903). The purpose of this chapter is not to add to the biographical research on Schreber, nor even to second-guess Freud. My intent is to provide a rereading of the *Memoirs* from the perspective of psychoanalytic self psychology, that is, from within the tradition originally articulated by Heinz Kohut (1971, 1977, 1984) and developed from the intersubjective perspective I share with Stolorow et al. (1987).

The first section of this chapter will provide a brief summary of Schreber's *Memoirs* and some biographical data; the second section will comment on Freud's account; and the third section will summarize some psychoanalytic contributions to the literature on Schreber since Freud. The chapter will focus on Schreber's self-experience from a relational–self-experience perspective. Almost every part of Schreber's self-experience consisted of his inference from, and organization of, his experience of being treated in particular ways by others. Recent research by psychoanalysts and historians supports more than a small developmental "kernel of truth" in Schreber's beliefs. In addition, Schreber clearly presented his delusions as his understanding of his treatment in the various asylums. "Here is what is happening to me," he seemed to say. Schreber wrote the *Memoirs* as an effort to organize and communicate his own experience so he could be found legally competent to manage his own affairs and to live outside the asylum. His book is the work of a judge writing to a judge, that is, by writing the book Schreber placed himself in an intersubjective field in which he could expect to find acknowledgment and respect. The final section of this chapter will examine this self-restorative process, the selfobject character of the book itself, and in particular the potential selfobject functions of the judge and court.

SCHREBER AND HIS MEMOIRS

Born in 1842, Daniel Paul Schreber, hereafter "Schreber," was the second son and third of five children born to Daniel Gottlob Moritz Schreber (from now on "Moritz Schreber") and Pauline Haase. Dr. Moritz Schreber, author of books on medical gymnastics and on childrearing practices, died when Schreber was 19 years old. Not much was known about Schreber's mother until Israels's (1989) biography of Schreber. It now appears that she was a major figure for Schreber until her death when he was in his 60s. Schreber became a jurist and rose quickly through the court system to become a prominent judge in Leipzig. He married in 1878, a year after his older brother, at age 38, committed suicide by gunshot. In 1885, Schreber became a candidate for the *Reichstag* (the imperial Diet, or legislature) from Chemnitz, where he held the post of *Landgerichtsdirektor,* the rank below president of the district court (Israels, 1989, p. 156). His first period of nervous disorder, as he termed it, or of hypochondria, as his psychiatrist Paul Emil Flechsig called it, occurred almost immediately after he lost this election. In the words of the clinic's psychiatric reports, "He imagines that he has lost thirty to forty pounds in weight. Has in fact gained two kilogrammes. Complains that he is being purposely deceived about his weight" (quoted in Baumeyer, 1956, pp. 61–62). By Schreber's (1903) own account, the first period passed "without any occurrences bordering on the supernatural" (p. 35). After 6 months in Flechsig's clinic in Leipzig, he returned to his wife and his work for 8 years. In 1893, he was appointed *Senatspraesident* in the *Oberlandsgericht* (superior court) in Dresden, and within weeks of taking up this position he was back in Flechsig's clinic for another 6 months. He was then transferred, after a 2-week stay in the Lindenhof clinic in Coswig, to the Sonnenstein public asylum at Pirna, near Dresden, for the following 8 years. The *Memoirs* chronicle this second period of illness. Schreber was released from Sonnenstein in 1902, but in 1907 after his mother's death, he became extremely agitated and was admitted to a clinic in Dosen, where he died in 1911.

Schreber began the *Memoirs* first, "to acquaint my wife with my personal experiences and religious ideas" so she would, after his release from Sonnenstein, be prepared to understand his "various oddities of behavior" (p. 1n). The project gradually gained, in his mind, a larger and larger intended audience. The expected readers expanded to include the courts that could find him competent to manage his own affairs and live outside the asylum, his former psychiatrist Flechsig, and finally an educated public who might find the work of scientific and religious value. Schreber's "personal experiences and religious ideas" became inextricably linked in his account because the religious ideas became his settled way of understanding and organizing his personal experiences. Nevertheless, for clarity, I will present his more-or-less straightforward narrative of his illness and treatment first.

After some general ideas about religious metaphysics and soul murder, Schreber began to tell his story:

> I will first consider some events *concerning other members of my family,* which may possibly be related to the presumed soul murder; these are all more or less mysterious, and can hardly be explained in the light of usual human experience (the further content of this chapter is omitted as unfit for publication). (p .61)

(The sections about Schreber's family had been censored before publication.) We are left to surmise what the rest of this chapter contained. Schreber's subsequent references to his family and to Flechsig usually spoke less directly about early ancestors of his relatives or of Flechsig.

Schreber then turned to the history of his illness. Within this account, he noted that just after his appointment as *Senatspraesident* he awoke one morning thinking "that it must really be rather pleasant to be a woman succumbing to intercourse" (p. 63). He also reported a sense of feeling burdened by his new position, in particular the need to earn the respect of the much older judges over whom he had to preside. He began to have difficulties sleeping, and he consulted Flechsig, who initially raised his hopes of a cure by prescribing sleeping drugs. When these did not work and Schreber looked for means of committing suicide, Flechsig advised Schreber to admit himself to Flechsig's asylum. The same pattern of the failure of sleeping drugs followed by suicide attempts recurred. Flechsig finally tried chloral hydrate as a sleeping aid. This treatment was successful, but Schreber's wife stopped visiting, and Flechsig, according to Schreber, could no longer look him straight in the eye when Schreber asked if he would recover. From then on, Schreber lived in a world of voices, divine miracles, and "fleeting-improvised" people, and he spent his days "bellowing" at God.

According to Schreber's account, he understood that the Order of the World had been disturbed and that he had to cooperate with God in resisting his own unmanning. He found, however, that his resistance was accompanied by divine interventions like the compression-of-the-chest-miracle, the writing-down-system, the appearance and disappearance of his stomach, the opening and closing of his eyes by miracles, the head-compressing machine, the coccyx miracle, which prevented him from staying in one place or position, the breaking of his piano strings, the system of unfinished sentences, and the constant torment of the voices.

Gradually Schreber became convinced that the way to make these tortures stop was to cooperate in his own transformation into a woman. He had to accept a completely passive role in his own life, thereby placating God, who, Schreber came to believe, was actually hostile to him. By accepting the sexual identity designated for him, he could redeem the world by giving birth to a new race.

FREUD'S ACCOUNT

Freud (1911) welcomed Schreber's *Memoirs* as a wonderful piece of evidence to support his own theory linking paranoia and homosexuality. As his title, "Psycho-Analytic Notes on an Autobiographical Account of a Case of Paranoia (Dementia Paranoides)," indicates, Freud saw Schreber as "a case of paranoia." Schreber was a clear confirmatory example of what Freud termed the "remarkable fact that the familiar principal forms of paranoia can all be represented as contradictions of the single proposition: 'I (a man) love him (a man)' " (p. 63). This theory-bound reading of the *Memoirs,* with Freud's propensity to exonerate fathers once he had minimized or disavowed the seduction theory (Bloch, 1989), undoubtedly shaped his understanding of Schreber. Nevertheless, Freud's essay contributed significantly to the understanding of the psychoses.

First and most important, Freud made the shift from symptom to meaning. Rejecting the psychiatric custom of inferring a diagnostic category from lists of symptoms, or of detailing delusions and concluding that the patient is insane, Freud insisted that symptoms and delusions have meaning. They refer, in other words, to something in the patient's experience or to the way the patient organizes experience. While Freud may have made gratuitous assumptions about the content and meaning of Schreber's experience—assumptions that probably limited his access to other meanings—still, he did consistently regard the psychoanalytic task as understanding the content and structure of the patient's subjective world.

More particularly, Freud saw Schreber's sense of being emasculated (his soul murder and self-loss) as central to his experience both of his threatened self and of the threatening others. Freud read "the end of the world" as referring to the destruction of Schreber's subjective world. Freud understood that the requirement that Schreber should redeem the world was a secondary, reactive, or even perhaps restorative aspect of his delusions. In addition, Freud (1911) saw Schreber's fear of sexual abuse as central to his experience and as probably involved in the "soul-murder" (p. 44). Freud was, however, unable to guess at any special reasons for Schreber's conviction that he was likely to be so abused.

Further, Freud clearly saw the parallels and identifications drawn by Schreber among God, Flechsig, and the sun—all three referred to Schreber's father—and Freud recognized Schreber's resulting mixture of hatred, love, and puzzlement toward them.

In fact, Freud was particularly well attuned to an important part of the subjective meaning of Schreber's belief that he must be transformed into a woman. Schreber was required to become a woman so he could feel like a woman—a person, in the eyes of both Freud and Schreber, who derives pleasure from being done to, from adopting a passive attitude, from submission. In addition, Freud and Schreber both saw female as equivalent to emasculated. Since Freud understood Schreber's God as his father, he thus recognized that Schreber felt compelled to take up a compliant passivity so extreme as to involve a change in physical sex characteristics. Because by this time Freud was locating pathology solely in the patient, he could not go further and ask what kind of childrearing might have produced the experience of such an extreme requirement of passivity or self-loss. Nor could Freud ask why the loss of selfhood—for Freud and Schreber, of masculinity—had to be accepted so completely that Schreber could no longer experience this loss as soul murder but had to feel it as redemptive.

Freud (1911) understood, however, just as I will argue in this chapter, that "the delusional formation, which we take to be the pathological product, is in reality an attempt at recovery, a process of reconstruction" (p. 71). Freud recognized, as did Schreber's physicians, that Schreber was more "sane" in his general behavior as his delusions became more fully articulated and organized. Finally, Freud saw the *Memoirs* as Schreber's attempt to rehabilite himself by trying to resolve his disputes with God/father. Freud (1911) commented on Dr. G. Weber's (director and chief psychiatrist of the Sonnenstein asylum) view that the *Memoirs* were "unblushing": "Surely we can hardly expect that a case history which sets out to give a picture of deranged humanity and its struggles to rehabilitate itself should exhibit 'discretion' and 'aesthetic' charm" (p. 37, n1).

Among the limitations of Freud's essay, already alluded to, is his method: the use of Schreber as a case to illustrate and support a theory, thus preventing Schreber from being seen as a person with a history of relationships reflected in the self-states described in the *Memoirs*. Freud's commitment to a one-person view of human nature and of psychopathology made it difficult, or perhaps impossible, for him to present Schreber's childhood or adult environments, including his treatment relationships, as structuring his inner world. Niederland (1984) would later view his researches into the work of Moritz Schreber as support for Freud's dynamic formulation. Still, Freud did not himself think it important to use in his account available information about either Schreber's family or about Flechsig's treatment philosophy. Nor did Freud, as far as we know, try to meet Schreber, who was still alive when Freud was writing about him. Perhaps this omission on Freud's part can be attributed to a concern that such researches would undermine or complicate his use of Schreber as a case to illustrate a one-person, instinct-based theory of paranoia.

We do have evidence that Freud thought about the effect of Schreber's early environment on him. Freud wrote to Ferenczi on October 6, 1910: "What would you think if old Dr. Schreber had worked 'miracles' as a physician? But was otherwise a tyrant in his household who 'shouted' [bellowed?] at his son and understood him as little as the 'lower God' understood our paranoiac" (Freud & Ferenczi, 1993, p. 222). We do not know why Freud chose to exclude these relational considerations from his published work on Schreber, but we can guess he found them inconsistent with his one-person view of psychopathology. If so, this omission illustrates my contention about the practical consequences of theory-choice and the importance of holding theory lightly.

Another limitation of Freud's essay on Schreber is that despite Freud's remarkable shift from symptom to meaning, he sometimes confused symbol and meaning, collapsing meaning into simple reference. He took symbols like unmanning as referring to castration, when Schreber made it clear that the much more serious and more real threat was soul murder or soul stealing. Stolorow et al. (1987) term such a collapse of meaning into symbol "concretization." Another example of confusing symbol and meaning in Freud's account—probably owing to his desire to support his own theory—is the assumption that Schreber transformed his father into God because "such a father as this was by no means unsuitable for transfiguration into a God in the affectionate memory of the son from whom he had been so early separated by death" (p. 51). Here

Freud saw the reference, or denotation, of the symbol but missed the emotional meaning. Schreber's God, a tyrant who regulates every part of life, was a tormentor. Freud recognized the distinction Schreber drew between Flechsig himself and "the Flechsig soul," between the objective and the subjective realities, and Freud knew each had a separate reference. Nevertheless, he bypassed the question of what experiential meaning Schreber's complaints against the Flechsig soul might carry. Freud apparently assumed that these were transference distortions of the behavior of an unequivocally benevolent physician. In addition, Freud saw Schreber's "megalomania" as compensatory for the insult of being turned into a woman. However, Freud missed—and here we cannot blame him for not seeing with Kohut's eyes—that the compensation in narcissistic grandiosity was for the complete self-loss that becoming a woman signified, a self-loss that had been required of him as a child.

A third limitation of Freud's interpretation, identifying the psychosis with an "outburst of homosexual libido," results from Freud's reliance on drive-theory assumptions about human motivation. Self psychologists instead attribute motivational primacy to self-consolidation—the need to organize emotional experience— and to relational concerns. Freud's Schreber, on the contrary, is a self-enclosed system of instinctual energy transformations. A related, though nonidentical, assumption—about homosexuality as one form of libido—led Freud to suggest that Schreber's psychosis manifested unconscious homosexuality, despite all evidence to the contrary. Schreber never behaved as a homosexual, nor is there any evidence that he thought of himself in that way. Freud, nevertheless, identified "feminine" and "homosexual" and took "it must be rather pleasant to be a woman succumbing to intercourse" Schreber, 1903, p. 63) as all the evidence he needed. For Freud, passivity or receptivity equals femininity, and femininity is equivalent, in a male, to homosexuality. Feeling attracted to same-sex partners is not required. As Lothane (1989) points out, Schreber gave no sign of sexual attraction to men. To Freud, this had to be unimportant: Homosexuality was an intrapsychic condition, not a relational matter.

Because of the limitations of his instinct theory, Freud also apparently missed the possibility that Schreber actually was persecuted and thus was not entirely delusional. (Freud, 1911, did, of course, insert his famous enigmatic caveat, "It remains for the future to decide whether there is more delusion in my theory than I should like to admit, or whether there is more truth in Schreber's delusion than other people are as yet prepared to believe" [p. 79], but he did not explore the implications of this statement.) Among those who have explored the possibilities, Lothane (1989) draws a convincing picture of the ways Schreber may have been mistreated by Flechsig. He construes Freud's reticence not only as political but as resulting from Freud's steadfast disinterest in the relational context of Schreber's difficulties.

Altogether, Freud's account directs us to the meanings in Schreber's psychosis, and then it systematically obscures these meanings. It has thus become the task of later psychoanalytic commentators and researchers to attempt to get closer to Schreber's own experience. Self psychology is especially well suited for this task because of its commitments to experience-near theorizing and to understanding the patient from the patient's point of view.

PSYCHOANALYTIC ACCOUNTS SINCE FREUD

Beginning with his 1951 paper "Three Notes on the Schreber Case" and continuing through the second edition of *The Schreber Case* (1984), Niederland provided the readers of Freud and Schreber with what he regarded as the "kernel of truth" in Schreber's complaints. His researches led him to believe that the "miracles" Schreber felt perpetrated on him were thinly veiled references to his father's childrearing methods. Niederland searched the books of Moritz Schreber and found pictures and descriptions of various pieces of apparatus—intended to correct improper posture or prevent its emergence—that seemed to resemble the "compression-of-the-chest-miracle," the "head-being-tied-together-machine," and others. He quoted extensive passages from Moritz Schreber's works that suggest an effort to control every part of a child's physical and mental life. In this way the child would develop so much self-control that he or she would not even feel externally coerced. No further discipline, according to Moritz Schreber, should be necessary after the fifth or sixth year of life. Niederland suggested that, like other 19th-century parents, Schreber's father's concern was to prevent children from masturbating. Niederland assembled a horrifying picture of the probable world of Schreber's childhood. This portrait not only makes his later fragmentation under stress understandable, and much detail of his report interpretable, but it also leaves the reader wondering how Schreber managed to function as long as he did. Niederland's book makes the older brother's suicide completely unsurprising.

What is surprising (to a reader unconcerned with protecting Freud and his theories) is that Niederland, having marshaled so much evidence of Schreber's persecutory childhood environment, nevertheless repeatedly and explicitly agreed with Freud's view of the case. Niederland concurred that Schreber was a "case of paranoia" to be explained in terms of intrapsychic conflict between love and hatred for the father, that is, rejection of his unconscious homosexual desire for the father and, later, for Flechsig. Niederland believed that his researches reinforced Freud's interpretation by showing that Schreber had reason to hate, and to love, his father and that the content of Schreber's *Memoirs* made even more sense than Freud had thought.

Niederland did not see that he had seriously undermined Freud's attempt to exonerate the father and place the cause of the paranoia solely in the patient. If the parallels Niederland drew are correct, early environment shaped Schreber's subjective world beyond any extent Freud was prepared to consider after he replaced the seduction theory. Niederland's relentless pursuit of historical meanings in Schreber's *Memoirs* makes his reluctance to draw the obvious conclusions from his own work puzzling.

Schatzman (1973) has no such hesitation. He, like Shengold (1989), straightforwardly accuses Moritz Schreber, with the full cooperation of his wife, of the soul murder, by prolonged physical and emotional abuse, of his sons. He agrees with Freud that the God of the *Memoirs* is Schreber's father, a deity who, Schreber only gradually comes to realize, intends to destroy his mind. Schatzman details, again by extensive reference to Moritz Schreber's books, the systematic ways the child, from infancy, is robbed of self-determination precisely under the rubric of self-determination. The child is programmed to want and not want precisely what the parents determine that the child should want and not want. This, to Schreber's father, is self-determination. (Schatzman provides a telling partial list of the titles of Moritz Schreber's books: *The Cold-Water Healing Method, The Systematically Planned Sharpening of the Senses,* and *The Harmful Body Positions and Habits of Children, Including a Statement of Counteracting Measures.*)

More recently, Lothane (1989, 1990), in the interpersonalist tradition, makes a strong case for regarding Schreber's psychosis as precipitated by his treatment by Flechsig and the other psychiatrists and by his wife's efforts to have him declared incompetent to manage his own affairs. Less convincing is Lothane's (1989) attempt "to vindicate both Schrebers, father and son" (p. 206). Lothane regards his own method as historical (fact not fancy) in contrast to what he sees as the hermeneutic or theory-bound method of Freud. He notes that the *Memoirs* seem to contain Schreber's account of what actually happened to him ("On the 1st of October 1893 I took up office as *Senatspraesident* to the Superior Court in Dresden") and his interpretation—cleverly disguised as delusional to avoid accusations of libel by Flechsig—of events ("Divine rays above all have the power of influencing the nerves"). Lothane apparently believes in a "just the facts" story about Schreber, as if any story could be told without interpretation or perspective (see Chapter 4). He thus dismisses the works of Niederland and Schatzman as "unproven inferences and constructions" (p. 209) and Freud's views as hermeneutics.

In Lothane's (1989, 1990) own interpretation of Schreber's story Schreber's psychosis was nondelusional; it was an extremely anxious response to his here-and-now situation, especially to his treatment by Flechsig. Agreeing with Schreber, Lothane believes that Flechsig committed soul murder on Schreber by assisting Schreber's wife in having him declared incompetent. According to Lothane, Flechsig thus "unmanned" Schreber by hypnotizing him, thereby robbing him of his reason, and by sending him to Sonnenstein, a public asylum for untreatable cases. Only then, according to Lothane, did Schreber's behavior become "insane." Schreber's diagnosis was, in this view, an iatrogenic psychosis. It is interesting, Lothane thinks, that Schreber never accused Weber, chief psychiatrist at Sonnenstein, of soul murder, even though Weber, according to Lothane, seriously mistreated Schreber by opposing his release when Schreber's behavior, by Weber's own account, had for a long time been reasonable, civil, and courteous.

Lothane's information about Flechsig, and his use of it to corroborate Schreber's statements in the "factual" parts of the *Memoirs,* is striking enough to make me wonder if more respectful treatment might not have prevented Schreber's full deterioration into a desperate, suicidal, bellowing madman who believed no one around him was real. Apparently Flechsig, a psychiatrist of his historical time, was interested only in biological treatments. What Lothane does not consider are the ways in which Schreber's early experience in his family preconditioned him to the experience of the stresses of his adult life—"overwork," Schreber called it—as well as to his mistreatment by Flechsig, Weber, and possibly his wife. Lothane is well aware of the intersubjective process in Schreber's treatment, but he misses the way a child may experience the relational world of the family and later find the adult world similar to that of childhood. In what follows, I will attempt to take the intersubjectively generated traumas of Schreber's childhood and his adulthood equally seriously. Schreber illustrates the clinical truism that abused children frequently become abused adults. What made Schreber extraordinary, besides Freud's interest in him, were his capacity and determination to tell his story and thus to heal himself by freeing himself from unjustified confinement.*

Kohut (1978a) wrote only briefly about Schreber. In Kohut's view, Freud's central insights in his writing on Schreber, were that " 'the *step back . . . to narcissism*' is characteristic of the psychoses, and that '*The delusional formation* . . . [is not the central pathology but] . . . *an attempt at recovery, a process of reconstruction . . .*' " (Kohut, 1978a, p. 306, quoting Freud, 1911, pp. 71–72). In his comments on Niederland's work on Moritz Schreber, Kohut remarked that the historical data could throw light on the essence of Schreber's psychosis: "the narcissistic fixation and regression" (p. 307). Kohut (1978a) believed that

> the secret of Schreber's psychosis is bound up with his father's personality—adding the important fact . . . that the mother was subordinated to, submerged by, and interwoven with the father's

---

*Without appropriate treatment, or other opportunities for substantial and primary selfobject experience, of course, his attempt at self-restoration was only partly and temporarily successful.

overwhelming personality and strivings, thus permitting the son no refuge from the impact of the father's pathology. (p. 307)

Kohut went on to explain that the father's pathology consisted of a special kind of psychotic character, in which reality-testing is generally present, but which, as in Hitler, is organized around a central *idée fixe*:

> The absolute conviction father Schreber had toward his ideas, the unquestioning fanaticism with which he pursued them, betrays, I believe, their profoundly narcissistic character, and I would assume that a fear of hypochondriacal tensions lies behind the rather overt fight against masturbation. His fanatical activities, too, although lived out on the body of the son, belong to a hidden narcissistic delusional system. The son, in other words, is felt as part of the father's narcissistic system, and not as separate. (p. 307)

Thus Kohut shifted the emphasis in understanding Schreber to the relational world of his childhood and to its bearing on his adult self-experience.

SCHREBER'S RELATIONAL EXPERIENCE

Schreber's self-experience, the primary concern of a self psychologically oriented analysis, can only be understood as the product of his experience of the intersubjective contexts, the emotional environments, in which he organized his sense of himself. While we have no direct access to the relational worlds of Schreber's childhood or adulthood, his *Memoirs* (1903) provide an eloquent account of his experience of and his interpretation of his psychiatric treatment. Without claiming to know the "facts" about either Schreber's childhood or about his treatment, we can consider the "organizing principles" (Stolorow et al., 1987) that he inferred from his relational experiences. This section will focus on the relational contexts in Schreber's life and Schreber's experience of them. The next section will attempt to describe Schreber's self-experience, its basis in his relational experiences, and its vicissitudes during the period covered by the *Memoirs*.

Schreber (1903) viewed his psychiatrist Flechsig and at least some of his caretakers as persecutors. He experienced them as attempting to murder his soul, to rob him of his reason, and to "unman" him for the sake of their own needs. He felt that they needed to get away from him because he was convinced that his needs, the "attraction of my nerves" (p. 128), were too much for the people around him. He thought that they gave him sleeping medicines so they could get away from him—not an implausible guess. They were, in other words, responding to their own needs, not to his.

> Always the main idea was to "forsake" me, that is to say, abandon me; at the times I am now discussing [just before he was sent away from Flechsig's asylum in 1894] it was thought that this could be achieved by unmanning me and allowing my body to be prostituted like that of a female harlot, sometimes also by killing me and later by destroying my reason (making me demented). (p. 99)

The beginning of this experience of persecution was a sense of being misunderstood. Early in November 1893, Schreber came to Flechsig complaining of sleeplessness and was given a combination of drugs that not only did not help him sleep but made him so anxious that he started to attempt suicide. By Schreber's account, the psychiatrists tried alternately to treat him with weaker sleeping drugs and with chloral hydrate, seeing his entire difficulty as a biologically based sleep disturbance. Each time the drugs failed, he tried to commit suicide. He felt that no attempt was made to understand him as an anxious living person:

> It is my opinion that Professor Flechsig must have had some idea of this tendency, innate in the Order of the World, whereby in certain conditions the unmanning of a human being is provided for. . . . A *fundamental misunderstanding* obtained, however, which has since run like a red thread through my entire life. It is based upon the fact *that within the Order of the World, God did not really understand the living human being* and had no need to understand him, because, according to the Order of the World, He dealt only with corpses. (p. 75)

> God . . . saw human beings *only from without*; as a rule his omnipresence and omniscience did not extend within *living* man. (pp. 59–60)

Schreber's indictment suggests that massive failures in empathic understanding, with a complete inattention to his subjective world, precipitated his turn from overwork and anxiety toward psychosis. God, Flechsig, and Moritz Schreber were devoted to an Order of the World, a scientific empiricism, in which the subjective world of the living human being could have no place. They could only comprehend beings with no feelings. Clearly Schreber meant in the quoted statements that he had never felt understood as a living human being with needs and feelings of his own, but had been seen, throughout his life, *"only from without."* He felt used and misunderstood by those who should have been his caretakers and protectors.

Once those others had misunderstood him, and classified him as a hopeless case, Schreber felt that they could and did abandon him. Once his wife, who had been visiting him daily, taking him out, and attempting to raise his spirits (p. 68), took a four-day vacation. He then had the night of "a quite unusual number of pollutions" (p. 68), which Freud took as an outburst of homosexual libido and Schreber understood as decisive in his deterioration. After that time he saw his wife rarely, experienced her as unreal, and began to talk instead with supernatural powers. He felt abandoned by everyone. No mention exists in any of his hospital records of any attempt by his wife, his mother, or his siblings to get him released from the hospital. The significance of the night of emissions, or "pollutions," may be that the combined abandonments meant complete loss of control: Moritz Schreber had believed that nocturnal emissions, and, of course, all masturbation, could and must be prevented.

Abandonment was also integral, not simply sequential, to the experience of misunderstanding. Misunderstanding of another can result from abandoning the subjective world, that is, the experience, of the patient or child. For Schreber, Flechsig's misunderstanding of him was experienced as so great an abandonment that he sometimes felt invisible: "something in the nature of a wizard had suddenly appeared in the person of Professor Flechsig . . . I myself, after all a person known in wider circles, had suddenly disappeared" (p. 97). At other times he felt that he must have leprosy, the disease of abandoned outcasts, or the plague. Later he felt required to think continuously, for fear God would misunderstand and regard "my mental powers as extinct" (p. 166). A partial function of the bellowing, paradoxically, was to interfere with God's abandonment of or withdrawal from him. It was both an indicator of madness and a cry for help. "It remains a riddle to me that the cries of help are apparently not heard by other human beings: the sound which reaches my own ear—hundreds of times every day—is so definite that it cannot be a hallucination" (p. 166). He was, however, deeply ashamed of his own needs. "The genuine 'cries of help' are always instantly followed by the phrase which has been learnt by rote: 'If only the cursed cries of help would stop' " (p. 166). We may speculate that in Schreber's family there had been no way for a child to cry for help. Both as a child and as a patient he felt abandoned, unsupported, and unvalidated (in his terms, misunderstood) in his extreme distress.

Schreber's sense of the total unreliability of others may be closely related to the experience of others as abandoning him. In the years before writing his account, Schreber felt that people do not even persist in being. They are *fluchtig hingemacht* (fleetingly made up), or, in Macalpine and Hunter's translation (Schreber, 1903), "cursorily improvised." People were not real; they were made-up contraptions. We can only speculate on the origins of this prominent feature of Schreber's experience of the human world. Perhaps Moritz Schreber's children never knew whether they would find him playful and affectionate or punitive and repressive. The father's books suggest that both attitudes are central to childrearing. Or perhaps Schreber's experience of his psychiatric treatment was that it included considerable improvisation and little consistency. Schreber may have experienced the massive unreliability in the environment as its unreality. Another possibility is that Schreber's upbringing deprived him of any sense of his own reality as a center of experience and initiative, which led him to say that others were unreal. If he is unreal so must others be. He may have felt himself to be a made-up contraption like the people in the illustrations in his father's books on medical gymnastics (cf. Niederland, 1984, pp. 81, 95). In any case, it is likely that Schreber's sense of the unreliability and unreality of human beings—particularly of those who should have been consistently helpful like his parents and physicians—contributed to his sense of abandonment, and the sense of abandonment, in turn, reinforced his sense that people were unreal and unreliable. Increasingly he understood both involvement with others and abandonment as intended to contribute to the destruction of his reason.

From misunderstanding and abandonment, soul murder continued to its central business of "unmanning." Lothane (1989) points out that, in German, "the word *Entmannung* has two basic meanings: the concrete one of gelding or castration, and the metaphorical one of loss of virile power, vigor, and pride" (p. 237). I agree with Lothane's view that Schreber consistently used the word in the second sense; I would add only that he felt the "loss" as a robbery and a betrayal. Consider the following:

> A plot was laid against me (perhaps March or April 1894), the purpose of which was to hand me over to another human being after my nervous illness had been recognized as, or assumed to be, incurable, in such a way that my soul was handed to him, but my body—transformed into a female body and, misconstruing the above-described fundamental tendency of the Order of the World—was then left to that human being for sexual misuse and simply "forsaken," in other words left to rot. (Schreber, 1903, p. 75)

Schreber's understanding of the intersubjective explanation for the efforts by others to murder his soul was that they saw him as a threat, as dangerous. He often spoke of the "miracles" directed against him as attempts to reduce his power to attract the nerves of God. He suspected that God—whom I take to stand for Moritz Schreber and, at times, Flechsig—had a manifest need to dominate, a need that covered a profound vulnerability. "God Himself must have been or be in a precarious position, if the conduct of a single human being could endanger Him in any way and if even He Himself, if only in lower instances, could be enticed into a kind of conspiracy against human beings who are fundamentally innocent" (p. 59). Parenthetically, this sense of being a threat to his older colleagues in his new position as *Senatspraesident* may have been one precipitant for his second period of illness. In Flechsig's clinic, he was likely to have questioned his treatment and thus seemed a threat to the established psychiatric hierarchy; as a child he may have known from experience that his father could not tolerate explicit or implicit questioning of his authority. Whatever the origins of this sense of others as threatened by his "nerves" (read as: feelings, needs, ideas), Schreber's conviction that others experienced him as dangerous runs throughout the *Memoirs*.

Another part of the soul murder was Schreber's sense of being used a guinea pig, a subject in endless experiments. Moritz Schreber supported his childrearing theories by claiming he had tested them on his own children. Flechsig probably tested his biological theories of psychiatry on the patients in his clinic. Schreber as patient thought he was surrounded by "tested souls." Experiments, of course, must be replicated: "God cannot learn by experience" (p. 155).

To be an experimental subject is, of course, not to be a person in one's own right, but to exist only to validate others' theories and to support the narcissistic needs of the experimenter. Schreber's primary complaint was that people attempted to destroy his reason and change his awareness of his own identity (p. 99), a common effect of childrearing by narcissistic parents (A. Miller, 1981).

The principal vehicle for the destruction of Schreber's soul or self, was, in his experience and expectation, sexual abuse. In his last months in Flechsig's clinic, "the most disgusting was the idea that my body, after the intended transformation into a female being, was to suffer some sexual abuse, particularly as there had even been talk for some time of my being thrown to the asylum attendants for this purpose" (p. 101). Now, whatever our estimate of the likelihood of sexual abuse of patients in Flechsig's clinic, Schreber's own sense of vulnerability and of being used was clearly tied to the experience of sexual abuse. He may have identified this vulnerability and the accompanying shame as equivalent to becoming female. If Schreber had been sexually abused as a child—possible in a family where children were experimental subjects—he would understandably experience any threat of sexual abuse as "unmanning," as depriving him of all autonomy, and as central to the stealing of his soul.

The sense of being used as an experimental subject may also have contributed to Schreber's messianic convictions. He believed God was creating a new race of humans out of his nerves, "new human beings out of Schreber's spirit" (p. 110). Moritz Schreber had had grandiose hopes for the improvement of the species by his childrearing methods, and he may have told his children of these dreams. For Schreber, as a mental patient, exposure to the experiment-over-treatment preference at Flechsig's clinic may have evoked a central organizing principle: transformation into a passive and vulnerable (i.e., female) person gives your life meaning— you contribute to the salvation of the world. Unmanning, he thought, might be "with the purpose of creating new human beings" (p. 117). Actively taking charge as *Senatspraesident* would have been too much opposed to this meaning, and it probably contributed to the evocation of his fantasy about how lovely being a woman passively succumbing to intercourse might be.

SCHREBER'S SELF-EXPERIENCE

Schreber's self-experience was organized by his relational experience both as a child and as an adult. His experience of persecution led him to see himself as dangerous to others and to explain the persecution and the miracles as attempts to control him because he was dangerous. His experience of what he called soul murder led him to experience himself as empty, both vulnerable and invulnerable (p. 212), helpless and unfree, unprotected (p. 117n), and female. Experience as an experimental subject led him to think of himself as important only if he could be used for some larger purpose like the salvation of the world. All these dimensions of his self-experience clearly emerged from his relational experiences as described above.

In addition, Schreber's self-experience was fragmented. He spoke of the partitioning of souls and of nerves strung out across the heavens, and he commented that he was inclined "to believe that the natural unity of the human soul used to be respected" (p. 109). His lack of cohesion displayed itself in his difficulty knowing who does the writing in the writing-down-system. He did not know how it came about that he was housed separately from the other patients; only later did he discover that it had been a response to his bellowing. The fragmentation was thus felt both as spatial and as temporal. Possibly because his relational experience had been traumatically inconsistent, and, perhaps, with Flechsig, desperately disappointing, he had considerable difficulty feeling himself as continuous in time. He reminds me of some highly intelligent and creative patients who protect themselves from overwhelming trauma through dissociation, with the resultant loss of continuity of experience of self and others. The confusion involved in such fragmentations may be integral to the soul murder process. Since the usurpation of the child's subjectivity is the essence of soul murder, Schreber had no basis for knowing anything. Schreber's self-experience during his confinements also took on an intensely negative coloration. Not only did he feel small, vulnerable (female), and without protection from the rays (p. 117n) but he also saw himself as stupid. Cognitively, he always knew that he had been a prominent judge, but this knowledge did nothing to hold at bay the voices that tormented him. When fellow patients would insult him, "the stupid twaddle of the voices 'has been recorded,' 'Why don't you say it (aloud)?', 'Because I am stupid,' or even 'Because I am afraid,' etc., tells me that it is still God's purpose that I relate these insulting forms of speech to myself" (pp. 199–200). He felt ashamed and humiliated by his condition and by his confinement. The voices often called him " 'wretch'—an expression quite common in the basic language to denote a human being destined to be destroyed by God and to feel God's power and wrath" (p. 124).

A particularly evocative expression of Schreber's negative self-valuation was his conviction during his first period of "nervous illness" that he had lost weight. To have weight, as philosopher Robert Nozick (1989) points out, is to be real and substantial, to have to be taken into account. In Nozick's words:

> The weight of something is its internal substantiality and strength. It may help to think of its opposite. What is meant when a person is called a "lightweight"? It might be impact and importance that are being talked about here, but usually, I think, what are meant are those qualities that importance is (or should be) based upon. People are commenting on how substantial the person is, how considered his thoughts, how dependable his judgment, how that person holds under buffeting or deeper examination. A weighty person is not blown by winds of fashion or scrutiny. The Romans called it *gravitas*. (p. 178)

This description probably fit Schreber the jurist well, and it points to the magnitude of the loss he felt.

The notion of weight is closely related to that of importance, which might be conceived as a more relational matter, that is, as having-weight-for-someone. In fact, Schreber's specific concern was about validation: "I believe I could have been more rapidly cured of certain hypochondriacal ideas with which I was preoccupied at the time, particularly concern over loss of weight, if I had been allowed to operate the scales which served to weigh patients a few times myself" (p. 62). For self psychologists, the self-experience of having weight, making a difference, would grow from the relational experience of having importance in the eyes of early caretakers and of having felt mirroring responses to one's own emerging selfhood. While we know that Moritz Schreber's children were important to him, from his writings we may infer that this importance resided in their value as experimental subjects and as exemplars of his childrearing methods. As mentioned above, he intended to eradicate every trace of the child's own will. The wishes and desires of children carried no weight with him, and his son, despite his impressive accomplishments, internalized a profound sense of himself as a lightweight. Schreber, as noted above, experienced himself and others as merely fleeting and improvised. As an asylum patient, the weightless Schreber was given to fits of bellowing, as if to impress his existence and presence—his weight—on his world and on God. For years, to experience himself as having any weight, he had to see others as fleeting-improvised Lilliputians. This view of the weight-loss experience may also lend intelligibility to Schreber's conviction that he was becoming a woman, a person of lesser weight and unimportant in 19th-century German society. He usually described his transformation into a woman as a process of shrinking. In his experience he replaced his quantitative loss (of weight) with a qualitative loss (of manhood).

Before we leave Schreber's self-experience as related in the *Memoirs,* we may note the absence of any obvious sadness in Schreber's words themselves. Schreber portrayed himself as feeling angry, humiliated, frustrated, abandoned, and destroyed, but never as sad. Perhaps sadness was the emotion that was thoroughly eradicated in his childhood by a constant demand to be cheerful. In addition, he may have had to ban this emotion from his repertoire in order not to suicide like his brother. In any case, his losses were considerable: home, wife, position and respect, autonomy, and peace of mind. Yet instead of feeling these losses, he said that he lost weight and masculinity.

SCHREBER'S EFFORTS AT SELF-RESTORATION

From the beginning of his illness, Schreber displayed a remarkable determination to restore, repair, and reclaim his stolen self. Not content with just surviving, he struggled to reestablish himself as a person of weight in his own eyes, in the eyes of God, and in the eyes of the human community. I will discuss his efforts in three categories: (1) his activities, (2) his paradoxical–passive efforts, and (3) the paranoia itself, seen as a self-reparative response to extreme narcissistic injury (soul murder).

Under the heading of activities, we may consider Schreber's piano-playing, chess-playing, learning of poetry, and, of course, his writing of the *Memoirs*. The first three activities were intended to convey to God, seen now as persecutor, that Schreber's soul had not been entirely destroyed. They also functioned to ward off the voices and miracles that otherwise tormented him.

The writing of the *Memoirs* was, however, the most direct of Schreber's efforts to restore himself to the status of a person in the human community. If Alice Miller (1990) is correct, abused children without a validating witness can neither experience their own pain, nor can they experience themselves as abused. Schreber was partly healed by his own process of attempting, by writing, to find such witnesses. He proclaimed both that he suffered and that crimes had been perpetrated on him. The probable reason that portions of his book were censored was that he had indicted his abusers by name, thereby claiming his own status as a human being. The *Memoirs* not only expressed his distress and outrage at the way he had been treated and at his own mental state, but it also signified his finding sufficient self-respect to challenge his tutelage. He overcame his feelings of weakness, helplessness, and shame enough to confront those who kept him in a less-than-human status. That he found the courage to engage in such an action of self-reclamation makes it probable that with adequate human support, he might have recovered faster, more thoroughly, and more permanently.

We can explain the restorative effect of writing the *Memoirs* by reference to the self psychological notion of selfobject experience. Even if primary selfobject relatedness is missing, anything can function as a selfobject to the extent that it contributes to the cohesiveness, continuity, and positive valence of a person's self-experience. For Schreber, the writing of his book apparently provided such derivative selfobject experience. By telling his story, even metaphorically, he attempted to make a coherent, continuous, and cohesive whole out of what felt absurd, confusing, and fragmenting. Both the story he told, and the action of telling it, transformed him from a bellowing madman into a learned, cultured, and genteel person who ate dinner and discussed various topics at the table of the director of the asylum. The story, submitted to the courts and to the director, also demanded recognition of the transformation. So not only did the act of writing serve as a selfobject experience for Schreber, but the book was clearly intended to evoke additional, even primary, selfobject experiences from his wife, the medical establishment, and the larger community.

Shifting now to Schreber's paradoxical–passive efforts at self-restoration, he also attempted from the time of his commitment to Sonnenstein to repair himself by surrendering to the requirements he felt had been placed on him. Literary critic E. Barry Chabot (1982) has pointed out a significant continuity among Schreber's desire to sleep, his catatonia, and his acceptance of the female "soul voluptuousness" (Schreber, p. 209). Each meant to him the possibility of release from torture by giving in to externally imposed requirements for the sake of a larger purpose. Initially, Schreber said that a person who could not sleep would surely have to suicide. Later he found that even with nocturnal sleep he was tormented by voices that demanded his complete immobility and by "miracles" that made every position he took, day or night, uncomfortable. (Schreber's father had invented devices and exercises to control children whether waking or sleeping.) Then for many months, the *Memoirs* inform us, Schreber sat for hours a day without moving. Finally he understood that God—not just "little Flechsig"—was tormenting him and demanding both his mental and physical passivity. Then he realized as well that he must actively cultivate the mental–physical state of female soul voluptuousness, the ultimate acquiescence. All three—sleep, catatonia, and soul voluptuousness—were perhaps attempts to rescue the self from torment. The last, however, became even temporarily healing when Schreber could understand its larger salvific meaning. Unfortunately he somehow, in the very acceptance of his passive role, both actively cooperated in his own destruction and rescued a vestige of himself, a kind of compromise sanity. We, of course, can see that this solution could not be stable for Schreber because it was based on compliance, on nonbeing, rather than on being a self. It was acceptance of the soul murder.

Finally Schreber's very paranoia may have been a prolonged effort at self-reparation. What he called soul murder was a lifelong narcissistic injury, an insult to the self, a cumulative trauma. His system of beliefs—delusions, many would call them—transformed his sense of vulnerability and stupidity into a grandiose belief that only he had access to ultimate religious truth. His helplessness became a power to attract the nerves of God. Confusion became a privileged access to meaning. His sense of profound insignificance became a mission to redeem the world precisely by adopting the role of insignificance assigned to women. A self psychological reading of Schreber must enthusiastically support Freud's (1911) view that "the delusional formation, which we take to be the pathological product, is in reality an attempt at recovery, a process of reconstruction" (p. 71).

Recognizing that Schreber did not simply write a summary of his delusions is important; he wrote his story with a beginning, a middle, and an ending. The beginning is lost to us because censors cut the sections referring to his family. The middle describes the miracles and other torments, along with Schreber's attempts to survive by resistance to the soul murder. His ending recounts the change, development, or transformation of his experience. By his account, once he accepted the fate dealt to him, he no longer found himself alone among cursorily improvised contraptions. He found other people real and himself significant. His book expresses Schreber's understanding of the process of what we can see as the temporary and partial restoration of his stolen self.

To summarize, Schreber's complaints fundamentally concern feeling profoundly misunderstood. His *Memoirs* was a plea for respectful understanding, an attempt to allow others to enter and share his emotional experience and to make sense of it with him. Faced instead with people who regarded him as a clinical case, he made his own case by writing for a court by which he hoped to be understood and restored to his status as a human being. Where he found the resources to imagine himself into such an intersubjective field we do not know, but his writing shows the power of the need for experienced understanding if a person is to be well.

The "Schreber case" also illustrates the influence of theory on our attempts to understand. If we refuse to do the hard work involved in conscious theory-choice, we leave ourselves to the control of unconscious, and thus unexamined, premises. In the story of Schreber, we can see the destructive power of uncritically held scientific empiricism (Schreber's father and Flechsig) and dogmatic instinct theory (Freud and Niederland). Further, even if we do consider and choose theory, we must hold it lightly. My own view of psychoanalytic understanding must remain provisional and open to surprise. Only so can I join the other in the healing process of making sense together.

References

Agosta, L. (1984). Empathy and intersubjectivity. In J. Lichtenberg, M. Bornstein, & D. Silver (Eds.), *Empathy I* (pp. 43–61). Hillsdale, NJ: The Analytic Press.

Alexander, F., & French, T. (1946). *Psychoanalytic Therapy: Principles and Application.* New York: Ronald Press.

Aquinas, T. (1265–1273). *The Summa Theologica,* Selections (English Dominican Fathers, Trans.). London: Everyman.

Aristotle (1941). Nicomachean ethics. In *The Basic Works of Aristotle* (R. McKeon, Ed.). New York: Random House.

Aron, L. (1991). The patient's experience of the analyst's subjectivity. *Psychoanalytic Dialogues, 1,* 29–51.

Aron, L. (1992). Interpretation as expression of the analyst's subjectivity. *Psychoanalytic Dialogues, 2,* 475–508.

Atwood, G., & Stolorow, R. (1984). *Structures of Subjectivity: Explorations in Psychoanalytic Phenomenology.* Hillsdale, NJ: The Analytic Press.

Atwood, G., & Stolorow, R. (1993). *Faces in a Cloud: Intersubjectivity in Personality Theory* (2nd ed.). Northvale, NJ: Jason Aronson.

Bacal, H. (1985). Optimal responsiveness and the therapeutic process. In A. Goldberg (Ed.), *Progress in Self Psychology* (Vol. 1, pp. 202–226). New York: Guilford Press.

Bacal, H. (1990). The elements of a corrective selfobject experience. *Psychoanalytic Inquiry, 10,* 347–372.

Bacal, H., & Newman, K. (1990). *Theories of Object Relations: Bridges to Self Psychology.* New York: Columbia University Press.

Bacal, H., & Thomson, P. (1993, October). *The psychoanalyst's needs and the effect of their frustration on the treatment: A new view of countertransference.* Paper presented at the Sixteenth Annual Conference on the Psychology of the Self, Toronto.

Balint, M. (1968). *The Basic Fault: Therapeutic Aspects of Regression.* Evanston, IL: Northwestern University Press, 1992.

Baumeyer, F. (1956). The Schreber case. *International Journal of Psycho-Analysis, 37,* 61–74.

Beebe, B., & Lachmann, F. (1988). Mother–infant mutual influence and precursors of psychic structure. In A. Goldberg (Ed.), *Frontiers in Self Psychology* (pp. 3–25). Hillsdale, NJ: The Analytic Press.

Beebe, B., & Lachmann, F. (1994). Representation and internalization in infancy: Three principles of salience. *Psychoanalytic Psychology, 11,* 127–165.

Bergson, H. (1910). *Time and Free Will* (F. Pogson, Trans.). New York: Harper Torchbooks, 1960.

Bernstein, R. (1983). *Beyond Objectivism and Relativism.* Philadelphia: University of Pennsylvania Press.

Bernstein, R. (1992). *The New Constellation: The Ethical–Political Horizons of Modernity/Postmodernity.* Cambridge, MA: MIT Press.

Bion, W. (1967). *Second Thoughts.* New York: Jason Aronson.

Bloch, D. (1989). Freud's retraction of his seduction theory and the Schreber case. *Psychoanalytic Review, 76,* 185–201.

Bollas, C. (1987). *The Shadow of the Object: Psychoanalysis of the Unthought Known.* London: Free Association Books.

Bollas, C. (1989). *Forces of Destiny: Psychoanalysis and Human Idiom.* London: Free Association Books.

Bowlby, J. (1979). *The Making and Breaking of Affectional Bonds.* London: Tavistock/Routledge.

Bowlby, J. (1988). *A Secure Base: Parent–Child Attachment and Healthy Human Development.* New York: Basic Books.

Brandchaft, B. (1983). The negativism of the negative therapeutic reaction and the psychology of the self. In A. Goldberg (Ed.), *The Future of Psychoanalysis* (pp. 327–359). New York: International Universities Press.

Brandchaft, B. (1985). Resistance and defense: An intersubjective view. In A. Goldberg (Ed.), *Progress in Self Psychology* (Vol. 1, pp. 88–96). New York: Guilford Press.

Brandchaft, B. (1986). British object relations and self psychology. In A. Goldberg (Ed.), *Progress in Seif Psychology* (Vol. 2, pp. 245–272). New York: Guilford Press.

Brandchaft, B. (1994, March). *Structures of pathological accommodation and change in analysis.* Paper presented at the meeting of the Association for Psychoanalytic Self Psychology, New York.

Breuer, J., & Freud, S. (1895). Studies on hysteria. *Standard Edition 2.* London: Hogarth Press, 1955.

Buber, M. (1937). *I and Thou.* Edinburgh, Scotland: T. & T. Clark.

Carnap, R. (1936). Testability and meaning. *Philosophy of Science, 3,* 419–471.

Chabot, E. (1982). *Freud on Schreber.* Amherst: University of Massachusetts Press.

Cohn, J., & Tronick, E. (1983). Three-month-old infants' reactions to simulated maternal depression. *Child Development, 54,* 185–193.

Cooper, S. (1993). Interpretive fallibility and the psychoanalytic dialogue. *Journal of the American Psychoanalytic Association, 41,* 95–126.

Copleston, F. (1950). *A History of Philosophy: Medieval Philosophy: Albert the Great to Duns Scotus.* Westminster, MD: Newman Press.

Courtois, C. (1988). *Healing the Incest Wound: Adult Survivors in Therapy.* New York: Norton.

Dilthey, W. (1989). *Introduction to the Human Sciences* (M. Neville, J. Barnouw, F. Schreiner, & R. Makkreel, Trans.). Princeton: Princeton University Press.

Eco, U. (1992). *Interpretation and Overinterpretation.* Cambridge, England: Cambridge University Press.

Ehrenberg, D. (1992). *The Intimate Edge: Extending the Reach of Psychoanalytic Interaction.* New York: Norton.

Ellenberger, H. (1970). *The Discovery of the Unconscious.* London: Penguin.

Emde, R. (1983). The prerepresentational self and its affective core. *Psychoanalytic Study of the Child, 38,* 165–192.

Emde, R. (1988a). Development terminable and interminable: I. Innate and motivational factors from infancy. *International Journal of Psycho-Analysis, 69,* 23–42.

Emde, R. (1988b). Development terminable and interminable: II. Psychoanalytic theory and therapeutic considerations. *International Journal of Psycho-Analysis, 69,* 283–296.

Emde, R., & Sorce, J. (1983). The rewards of infancy: Emotional availability and maternal referencing. In J. Call, E. Galenson, & R. Tyson (Eds.), *Frontiers of Infant Psychiatry* (pp. 17–30). New York: Basic Books.

Fairbairn, W. (1952). *Psychoanalytic Studies of the Personality.* London: Tavistock/Routledge and Kegan Paul.

Ferenczi, S. (1909). Stages in the development of a child's sense of reality. In *First Contributions to Psycho-Analysis* (E. Jones, Trans.; pp. 102–107). London: Hogarth Press, 1952.

Ferenczi, S. (1929). The unwelcome child and his death instinct. In *Final Contributions to the Problems and Methods of Psycho-Analysis* (M. Balint, Ed.; pp. 102–107). New York: Brunner/Mazel, 1955.

Ferenczi, S. (1932). Notes and fragments. In *Final Contributions to the Problems and Methods of Psycho-Analysis* (M. Balint, Ed.; pp. 216–278), New York: Brunner/Mazel, 1955.

Ferenczi, S. (1933). The confusion of tongues between adults and the child. In *Final Contributions to the Problems and Methods of Psycho-Analysis* (M. Balint, Ed.; pp. 156–167). New York: Brunner/Mazel, 1955.

Ferenczi, S. (1988). *The Clinical Diaries of Sandor Ferenczi.* Cambridge, MA: Harvard University Press.

Flavell, J. (1977). *Cognitive Development.* Englewood Cliffs, NJ: Prentice Hall.

Fosshage, J. (1992a, April). *Countertransference as the analyst's experience of the analysand: The influence of listening perspectives.* Paper presented at the meeting of the Division of Psychoanalysis of the American Psychological Association, Philadelphia.

Fosshage, J. (1992b). Self psychology: The self and its vicissitudes within a relational matrix. In N. Skolnick & S. Warshaw (Eds.), *Relational Perspectives in Psychoanalysis* (pp. 21–42). Hillsdale, NJ: The Analytic Press.

Fosshage, J. (1994). Towards reconceptualizing transference: Theoretical and clinical considerations. *International Journal of Psycho-Analysis, 75,* 265–280.

Freud, A. (1936). *The Ego and the Mechanisms of Defense.* New York: International Universities Press, 1966.

Freud, S. (1895). Project for a scientific psychology. *Standard Edition 1* (pp. 283–397). London: Hogarth Press, 1950.

Freud, S. (1910). Five lectures on psycho-analysis. *Standard Edition, 11* (pp. 9–55). London: Hogarth Press, 1957.

Freud, S. (1911). Psycho-analytic notes on an autobiographical account of a case of paranoia (dementia paranoides). *Standard Edition 12* (pp. 3–82). London: Hogarth Press, 1958.

Freud, S. (1912). Recommendations to physicians practising psycho-analysis. *Standard Edition 12* (pp. 109–120). London: Hogarth Press, 1958.

Freud, S. (1914). Remembering, repeating and working through. *Standard Edition 12* (pp. 145–156). London: Hogarth Press, 1958.

Freud, S. (1919). Preface to Reik's *Ritual: Psycho-Analytic Studies. Standard Edition 17* (pp. 259–263). London: Hogarth Press, 1955.

Freud, S. (1925). Some psychical consequences of the anatomical distinction between the sexes. *Standard Edition 19* (pp. 243–258). London: Hogarth Press, 1961.

Freud, S., & Ferenczi, S. (1993). *The Correspondence of Sigmund Freud and Sandor Ferenczi: Vol. 1. 1908–1914* (E. Brabant, E. Falzeder, & P. Gampieri-Deutsch, Eds., P. Hoffer, Trans.). Cambridge, MA: Harvard University Press.

Fromm-Reichmann, F. (1950). *Principles of Intensive Psychotherapy.* Chicago: University of Chicago Press.

Gadamer, H. (1976). *Philosophical Hermeneutics* (D. Linge, Trans.). Berkeley: University of California Press.

Gadamer, H. (1979). The problem of historical consciousness. In P. Rabinow & W. Sullivan (Eds.), *Interpretive Social Science: A Reader.* Berkeley: University of California Press.

Gadamer, H. (1991). *Truth and Method* (2nd ed., J. Weinsheimer & D. Marshall, Trans.). New York: Crossroads.

Geha, R. (1993). Transferred fictions. *Psychoanalytic Dialogues, 3,* 209–244.

Gerson, M. (1993). Sullivan's self-in-development: Family context and patterning. *Contemporary Psychoanalysis, 29,* 197–218.

Ghent, E. (1992). Paradox and process. *Psychoanalytic Dialogues, 2,* 135–159.

Gill, M. (1982). *Analysis of Transference* (Vol. 1). New York: International Universities Press.

Goldberg, A. (1988). *A Fresh Look at Psychoanalysis: The View from Self Psychology.* Hillsdale, NJ: The Analytic Press.

Gotthold, J. (1992, October). *Curative fantasy: Its function in the treatment process.* Paper presented at the Fifteenth Annual Conference on the Psychology of the Self, Los Angeles.

Greenberg, J. (1991). *Oedipus and Beyond.* Cambridge, MA: Harvard University Press.

Greenberg, J. (1992). Developmental perspectives in psychoanalytic practice: Panel discussion. *Contemporary Psychoanalysis, 28,* 251–299.

Greenberg, J., & Mitchell, S. (1983). *Object Relations in Psychoanalytic Theory.* Cambridge, MA: Harvard University Press.

Grosskurth, P. (1987). *Melanie Klein: Her World and Her Work.* Cambridge, MA: Harvard University Press.

Grunbaum, A. (1984). *The Foundations of Psychoanalysis: A Philosophical Critique.* Berkeley: University of California Press.

Guntrip, H. (1969). *Schizoid Phenomena, Object Relations and the Self.* New York: International Universities Press.

Hanly, C. (1992). *The Problem of Truth in Applied Psychoanalysis.* New York: Guilford Press.

Hegel, G. (1807). *Phenomenology of Spirit* (A. Miller, Trans.). Oxford, England: Oxford University Press, 1977.

Hempel, C. (1951). The concept of cognitive significance: A reconsideration. *Proceedings of the American Academy for the Advancement of Science, 80,* 61–77.

Herman, J. L. (1992). *Trauma and Recovery.* New York: Basic Books.

Hesse, M. (1980). *Revolutions and Reconstructions in the Philosophy of Science.* Brighton, England: Harvester Press.

Hobson, R. F. (1985). *Forms of Feeling: The Heart of Psychotherapy.* London: Tavistock.

Hoffman, I. (1983). The patient as interpreter of the analyst's experience. *Contemporary Psychoanalysis, 19,* 389–422.

Hoffman, I. (1987). The value of uncertainty in psychoanalytic practice. *Contemporary Psychoanalysis, 23,* 205–215.

Hoffman, I. (1991). Discussion: Toward a social-constructivist view of the psychoanalytic situation. *Psychoanalytic Dialogues, 1,* 74–105.

Hoffman, I. (1992a). Reply to Orange. *Psychoanalytic Dialogues, 2,* 567–570.

Hoffman, I. (1992b). Some practical implications of a social-constructivist view of the psychoanalytic situation. *Psychoanalytic Dialogues, 2,* 287–304.

Hoffman, I. (1993). The intimate authority of the psychoanalyst's presence. *Psychologist Psychoanalyst, 13,* 15–23.

Horowitz, M. (1986). *Stress Response Syndromes* (2nd ed.). Northvale, NJ: Jason Aronson.

Hume, D. (1739). *A Treatise of Human Nature.* Oxford, England: Oxford University Press, 1896.

Husserl, E. (1931). *Ideas: An Introduction to Pure Phenomenology.* New York: Macmillan.

Israels, H. (1989). *Schreber: Father and Son.* Madison, CT: International Universities Press.

Jaenicke, C. (1987). Kohut's concept of cure. *Psychoanalytic Review, 74,* 537–548.

James, W. (1892). *Textbook of Psychology: Briefer Course.* New York: Holt.

James, W. (1902). *The Varieties of Religious Experience.* London: Longmans Green.

James, W. (1905). The place of affectional facts in a world of pure experience.

In *Essays in Radical Empiricism* (R. Perry, Ed.; pp. 72–80). New York: Dutton, 1971.

James, W. (1907). *Pragmatism.* Cambridge, MA: Harvard University Press, 1975.

James, W. (1909). *The Meaning of Truth.* Cambridge, MA: Harvard University Press, 1975.

Jones, J. (1995). *Affects as Process: An Inquiry into the Centrality of Affect in Psychological Life.* Hillsdale, NJ: The Analytic Press.

Kant, I. (1781). *Critique of Pure Reason* (N. Kemp Smith, Trans.). New York: Macmillan, 1929.

Kernberg, O. (1986). Factors in the psychoanalytic treatment of narcissistic personalities. In A. Morrison (Ed.), *Essential Papers on Narcissism* (pp. 213–244). New York: New York University Press.

Kirk, G., & Raven, S. (1984). *The Presocratic Philosophers: A Critical History with a Selection of Texts* (2nd ed.). Cambridge, England: Cambridge University Press.

Klein, G. (1966). *Perception, Motives and Personality.* New York: Knopf.

Klein, G. (1976). *Psychoanalytic Theory.* New York: International Universities Press.

Klein, M. (1975). *Envy and Gratitude, 1946–1963.* New York: Delacorte Press.

Kohut, H. (1957). Observations on the psychological functions of music. In *The Search for the Self* (Vol. 1, P. Ornstein, Ed.; pp. 233–253). Madison, CT: International Universities Press, 1978.

Kohut, H. (1959). Introspection, empathy, and psychoanalysis: An examination of the relationship between mode of observation and theory. In *The Search for the Self* (Vol. 1, P. Ornstein, Ed.; pp. 205–232). Madison, CT: International Universities Press, 1978.

Kohut, H. (1971). *The Analysis of the Self.* New York: International Universities Press.

Kohut, H. (1973). The psychoanalyst in the community of scholars. In *The Search for the Self* (Vol. 2, P. Ornstein, Ed.; pp. 685–724). Madison, CT: International Universities Press, 1978.

Kohut, H. (1977). *The Restoration of the Self.* Madison, CT: International Universities Press.

Kohut, H. (1978a). Discussion of "Further data and documents in the Schreber case" by William G. Niederland. In *The Search for the Self* (Vol. 1, P. Ornstein, Ed.; pp. 305–308). Madison, CT: International Universities Press.

Kohut, H. (1978b). Conclusion: The search for the analyst's self. In *The Search for the Self* (Vol. 2, P. Ornstein, Ed.; pp. 931–938). Madison, CT: International Universities Press.

Kohut, H. (1978c). Letter to a colleague. In *The Search for the Self* (Vol. 4, P. Ornstein, Ed.; pp. 577–591). Madison, CT: International Universities Press, 1991.

Kohut, H. (1981). On empathy. In *The Search for the Self* (Vol. 4, P. Ornstein, Ed.; pp. 525–535). Madison, CT: International Universities Press, 1991.

Kohut, H. (1984). *How Does Analysis Cure?* Chicago: University of Chicago Press.

Kohut, H. (1985). *Self Psychology and the Humanities: Reflections on a New Psycho-analytic Approach* (C. Strozier, Ed.). New York: Norton.

Kohut, H. (1994). *The Curve of Life: Correspondence of Heinz Kohut, 1923–1981* (G. Cocks, Ed.). Chicago: University of Chicago Press.

Krystal, H. (1988). *Integration and Self-Healing: Affect, Trauma, Alexithymia.* Hillsdale, NJ: The Analytic Press.

Kuhn, T. (1962). *The Structure of Scientific Revolutions* (2nd ed.). Chicago: University of Chicago Press, 1970.

Lauer, Q. (1976). *A Reading of Hegel's* Phenomenology of Spirit. New York: Fordham University Press.

Lauer, Q. (1978). *The Triumph of Subjectivity: An Introduction to Transcendental Phenomenology.* New York: Fordham University Press.

Lessem, P. (1992, October). *The relational patterning of affective experience.* Paper presented at the Fifteenth Annual Conference on the Psychology of the Self, Los Angeles.

Lessem, P., & Orange, D. (1993, October). *Self psychology and attachment: The importance of the particular other.* Paper presented at the Sixteenth Annual Conference on the Psychology of the Self, Toronto.

Lichtenberg, J. (1983). *Psychoanalysis and Infant Research.* Hillsdale, NJ: The Analytic Press.

Lichtenberg, J. (1989). *Psychoanalysis and Motivation.* Hillsdale, NJ: The Analytic Press.

Lichtenberg, J., Lachmann, F., & Fosshage, J. (1993). *Self and Motivational Systems: Toward a Theory of Psychoanalytic Technique.* Hillside, NJ: The Analytic Press.

Little, M. (1990). *Psychotic Anxieties and Containment: A Personal Record of an Analysis with Winnicott.* Northvale, NJ: Jason Aronson.

Loewald, H. (1960a). On the therapeutic action of psychoanalysis. *International Journal of Psycho-Analysis, 41,* 16–33.

Loewald, H. (1960b). Perspectives on memory. In *Papers on Psychoanalysis.* New Haven, CT: Yale University Press, 1980.

Loewald, H. (1980). *Papers on Psychoanalysis.* New Haven, CT: Yale University Press.

Loewald, H. (1986). Transference–countertransference. *Journal of the American Psychoanalytic Association, 34,* 275–287.

Lomas, P. (1987). *The Limits of Interpretation.* Northvale, NJ: Jason Aronson.

Lothane, Z. (1989). Schreber, Freud, Flechsig and Weber revisited: An inquiry into methods of interpretation. *Psychoanalytic Review, 76,* 203–262.

Lothane, Z. (1990). [Panel on Schreber at the American Academy of Psychoanalysis.] On tape.

Maccio, D. (1992). Surviving, existing, living: Reflections on the analyst's anxiety. In L. Nissim-Momigliano & A. Robutti (Eds.), *Shared Experience* (pp. 89–120). London: Karnac Books.

Macmurray, J. (1957). *The Self as Agent.* Atlantic Highlands, NJ: Humanities Press International, 1991.

Magid, B. (Ed.). (1993). *Freud's Case Studies: Self Psychological Perspectives.* Hillsdale, NJ: The Analytic Press.

Mahler, M., Pine, F., & Bergman, A. (1975). *The Psychological Birth of the Human Infant.* New York: Basic Books.

McDougall, J. (1989). *Theaters of the Body: A Psychoanalytic Approach to Psychosomatic Illness.* New York: Norton.

Miller, A. (1981). *Prisoners of Childhood* (R. Ward, Trans.). New York: Basic Books.

Miller, A. (1986). Depression and grandiosity as related forms of narcissistic disturbances. In A. Morrison (Ed.), *Essential Papers on Narcissism* (pp. 323–347). New York: New York University Press.

Miller, A. (1990). *The Untouched Key: Tracing Childhood Trauma in Creativity and Destructiveness* (H. Hannum & H. Hannum, Trans.). New York: Doubleday Anchor Books.

Miller, J., & Post, S. (Eds.). (1990). How theory shapes technique: Perspectives on a self psychological clinical presentation. *Psychoanalytic Inquiry, 10,* (459–624).

Mitchell, S. (1988). *Relational Concepts in Psychoanalysis: An Integration.* Cambridge, MA: Harvard University Press.

Mitchell, S. (1993). *Hope and Dread in Psychoanalysis.* New York: Basic Books.

Moore, B., & Fine, R. (1990). *Psychoanalytic Terms and Concepts.* New Haven, CT: Yale University Press.

Niederland, W. (1951). Three notes on the Schreber case. *Psychoanalytic Quarterly, 28,* 151–169.

Niederland, W. (1984). *The Schreber Case* (2nd ed.). Hillsdale, NJ: The Analytic Press.

Nissim-Momigliano, L., & Robutti, A. (Eds.). (1992). *Shared Experience.* London: Karnac Books.

Nozick, R. (1989). *The Examined Life.* New York: Simon and Schuster.

Nozick, R. (1993). *The Nature of Rationality.* Princeton: Princeton University Press.

Ogden, T. (1986). *The Matrix of the Mind.* Northvale, NJ: Jason Aronson.

Ogden, T. (1989). *The Primitive Edge of Experience.* Northvale, NJ: Jason Aronson.

Ogden, T. (1994). *The Subjects of Analysis.* Northvale, NJ: Jason Aronson.

Orange, D. (1984). *Peirce's Conception of God.* Bloomington: Indiana University Press.

Orange, D. (1992a). Commentary on Irwin Hoffman's "Discussion: Toward a social constructivist view of the psychoanalytic situation." *Psychoanalytic Dialogues, 2,* 561–566.

Orange, D. (1992b). Subjectivism, relativism, and realism in psychoanalysis. In A. Goldberg (Ed.), *New Therapeutic Visions: Progress in Self Psychology* (pp. 189–197). Hillsdale, NJ: The Analytic Press.

Orange, D. (1993). The restoration of Schreber's stolen self. In B. Magid (Ed.), *Freud's Case Studies: Self Psychological Perspectives.* Hillsdale, NJ: The Analytic Press.

Orange, D. (1994). Countertransference, empathy, and the hermeneutical circle. In R. Stolorow, G. Atwood, & B. Brandchaft (Eds.), *The Intersubjective Perspective* (pp. 177–186). Northvale, NJ: Jason Aronson.

Orange, D. (1995, April). *Relationship theories and self psychology: The Ferenczi connection.* Paper presented at the meeting of the Division of Psychoanalysis of the American Psychological Association, Santa Monica, CA.

Ornstein, A. (1991). The dread to repeat: Comments on the working through process in psychoanalysis. *Journal of the American Psychoanalytic Association, 39,* 377–398.

Ornstein, P. (1991). Why self psychology is not an object relations theory: Clinical and theoretical considerations. In A. Goldberg (Ed.), *The Evolution of Self Psychology: Progress in Self Psychology* (pp. 17–29). Hillsdale, NJ: The Analytic Press.

Ornstein, P., & Ornstein, A. (1985). Clinical understanding and explaining: The empathic vantage point. In A. Goldberg (Ed.), *Progress in Self Psychology* (Vol. 1, pp. 43–61). New York: Guilford Press.

Palmer, R. (1969). *Hermeneutics: Interpretation Theory in Schleiermacher, Dilthey, Heidegger, and Gadamer.* Evanston, IL: Northwestern University Press.

Peirce, C. (1868). Some consequences of four incapacities. In *Collected Papers of Charles Sanders Peirce* (Vol. 5, C. Hartshorne & P. Weiss, Eds.; pp. 156–189). Cambridge, MA: Harvard University Press, 1931–1935.

Peirce, C. (1877). The fixation of belief. In *Collected Papers of Charles Sanders Peirce* (Vol. 5, C. Hartshorne & P. Weiss, Eds.; pp. 223–247). Cambridge, MA: Harvard University Press, 1931–1935.

Peirce, C. (1931–1935). *Collected Papers of Charles Sanders Peirce* (C. Hartshorne & P. Weiss, Eds.). Cambridge, MA: Harvard University Press.

Piaget, J. (1968). *On the Development of Memory and Identity.* Barre, MA: Clark University Press and Barre Publishers.

Piaget, J., & Inhelder, B. (1973). *Memory and Intelligence.* New York: Basic Books.

Pine, F. (1990). *Drive, Ego, Object, and Self.* New York: Basic Books.

Plato (1961). *Collected Dialogues.* Princeton, NJ: Princeton University Press.

Polanyi, M. (1958). *Personal Knowledge: Towards a Post-Critical Philosophy.* Chicago: University of Chicago Press.

Popper, K. (1959). *The Logic of Scientific Discovery.* New York: Harper & Row.

Potter, V. (1994). *On Understanding Understanding.* New York: Fordham University Press.

Protter, B. (1985). Toward an emergent psychoanalytic epistemology. *Contemporary Psychoanalysis, 21,* 208–227.

Pulver, S. (Ed.). (1987). Models of the mind: Perspectives on a clinical study. *Psychoanalytic Inquiry, 7,* 141–299.

Racker, H. (1968). *Transference and Countertransference.* New York: International Universities Press.

Renik, O. (1993). Analytic interaction: Conceptualizing technique in light of the analyst's irreducible subjectivity. *Psychoanalytic Quarterly, 62,* 553–571.

Ricci, W., & Broucek, F. (1994, October). *Neutrality, abstinence and anonymity revisited.* Paper presented at the Seventeenth Annual Conference of the Psychology of the Self, Chicago.

Ricoeur, P. (1979). The model of the text: Meaningful action considered as a text. In P. Rabinow & W. Sullivan (Eds.), *Interpretive Social Science: A Reader* (pp. 73–101). Berkeley: University of California Press.

Rilke, R. (1934). *Letters to a Young Poet.* New York: Norton.

Ryle, G. (1949). *The Concept of Mind.* London: Hutchinson.

Schachtel, E. (1959). *Metamorphosis.* New York: Basic Books.

Schafer, R. (1983). *The Analytic Attitude.* New York: Basic Books.

Schatzman, M. (1973). *Soul Murder: Persecution in the Family.* New York: Random House.

Schreber, D. (1903). *Memoirs of My Nervous Illness* (I. Macalpine & R. Hunter, Eds. & Trans.). Cambridge, MA: Harvard University Press, 1955.

Schwaber, E. (1983). Construction, reconstruction, and the mode of clinical attunement. In A. Goldberg (Ed.), *The Future of Psychoanalysis* (pp. 273–291). New York: International Universities Press.

Schwaber, E. (1992). Countertransference: The analyst's retreat from the patient's vantage point. *International Journal of Psycho-Analysis, 73,* 349–362.

Shabad, P. (1993). Resentment, indignation, entitlement: The transformation of unconscious wish into need. *Psychoanalytic Dialogues, 3,* 481–494.

Shengold, L. (1989). *Soul Murder: The Effects of Childhood Abuse and Deprivation.* New Haven, CT: Yale University Press.

Spence, D. (1982). *Narrative Truth and Historical Truth.* New York: Norton.

Spezzano, C. (1993). *Affect in Psychoanalysis: A Clinical Synthesis.* Hillsdale, NJ: The Analytic Press.

Spiegelberg, H. (1960). *The Phenomenological Movement* (Vols. 1–2). The Hague, The Netherlands: Martinus Nijhoff.

Spinoza, B. (1677). *Ethics.* New York: Hafner, 1949.

Stern, Daniel (1983). Implications of infancy research for psychoanalytic theory and practice. *Psychiatric Update, 2,* 7–21.

Stern, Daniel (1985). *The Interpersonal World of the Infant.* New York: Basic Books.

Stern, Daniel (1988). The dialectic between the "interpersonal" and the "intrapsychic": With particular emphasis on the role of memory and representation. *Psychoanalytic Inquiry, 8,* 505–512.

Stern, Donnel. (1989). The analyst's unformulated experience of the patient. *Contemporary Psychoanalysis, 25,* 1–33.

Stern, Donnel. (1991). A philosophy for the embedded analyst: Gadamer's hermeneutics and the social paradigm of psychoanalysis. *Contemporary Psychoanalysis, 27,* 51–58.

Stern, Donnel. (1992). Commentary on constructivism in clinical psychoanalysis. *Psychoanalytic Dialogues, 2,* 331–363.

Stolorow, D., & Stolorow, R. (1987). Affects and selfobjects. In R. Stolorow, B. Brandchaft, & G. Atwood, *Psychoanalytic Treatment: An Intersubjective Approach* (pp. 66–87). Hillsdale, NJ: The Analytic Press.

Stolorow, R. (1988). Intersubjectivity, psychoanalytic knowing, and reality. *Contemporary Psychoanalysis, 24,* 331–338.

Stolorow, R. (1994). The nature and therapeutic action of psychoanalytic interpretation. In R. Stolorow, G. Atwood, & B. Brandchaft (Eds.), *The Intersubjective Perspective* (pp. 43–55). Northvale, NJ: Jason Aronson.

Stolorow, R., & Atwood, G. (1992). *Contexts of Being: The Intersubjective Foundations of Psychological Life.* Hillsdale, NJ: The Analytic Press.

Stolorow, R., Brandchaft, B., & Atwood, G. (1987). *Psychoanalytic Treatment: An Intersubjective Approach.* Hillsdale, NJ: The Analytic Press.

Stolorow, R., & Lachmann, F. (1987). Transference—The organization of experience. In R. Stolorow, B. Brandchaft, & G. Atwood, *Psychoanalytic Treatment: An Intersubjective Approach* (pp. 28–46). Hillsdale, NJ: The Analytic Press.

Strachey, J. (1934). The nature of the therapeutic action of psychoanalysis. *International Journal of Psycho-Analysis, 15,* 127–159.

Sucharov, M., (1994). Psychoanalysis, self psychology, and intersubjectivity. In R. Stolorow, G. Atwood, & B. Brandchaft (Eds.), *The Intersubjective Perspective* (pp. 187–202). Northvale, NJ: Jason Aronson.

Sullivan, H. (1940). *Conceptions of Modern Psychiatry.* New York: Norton.

Sullivan, H. (1953). *The Interpersonal Theory of Psychiatry.* New York: Norton.

Sulloway, F. (1979). *Freud, Biologist of the Mind: Beyond the Psychoanalytic Legend.* New York: Basic Books.

Suppe, F. (1977). *The Structure of Scientific Theories* (2nd ed.). Urbana: University of Illinois Press.

Suttie, I. (1935). *The Origins of Love and Hate.* London: Routledge and Kegan Paul, 1988.

Tansey, M. (1992). Psychoanalytic expertise. *Psychoanalytic Dialogues, 2,* 305–316.

Tauber, E., & Green, M. (1959). *Prelogical Experience.* New York: Basic Books.

Terr, L. (1990). *Too Scared to Cry.* New York: HarperCollins.

Thomson, P. (1991). Countertransference in an intersubjective perspective: An experiment. In A. Goldberg (Ed.), *The Evolution of Self Psychology* (pp. 75–92). Hillsdale, NJ: The Analytic Press.

Tolpin, M. (1991). Conversations. In J. Masterson, M. Tolpin, & P. Sifneos (Eds.), *Comparing Psychoanalytic Psychotherapies.* New York: Brunner/Mazel.

Tomkins, S. (1963). *Affect, Imagery, Consciousness, II: The Negative Affects.* New York: Springer.

Tronick, E. (1989). Emotions and emotional communication in infants. *American Psychologist, 44,* 112–119.

van der Kolk, B. (1984). *Post-Traumatic Stress Disorder: Psychological and Biological Sequelae.* Washington, DC: American Psychiatric Press.

van der Kolk, B. (1987). *Psychological Trauma.* Washington, DC: American Psychiatric Press.

Waelder, R. (1936). The principle of multiple function. *Psychoanalytic Quarterly, 15,* 45–62.

Wallerstein, R. (Ed.). (1992). *The Common Ground of Psychoanalysis.* Northvale, NJ: Jason Aronson.

Weigert, E. (1962). Sympathy, empathy, and freedom in therapy. In L. Salzman & J. Masserman (Eds.), *Modern Concepts of Psychoanalysis.* New York: Citadel Press.

Whitehead, A. N. (1925). *Science and the Modern World.* New York: Macmillan.

Whitehead, A. N. (1929). *Process and Reality.* New York: Macmillan.

Whitehead, A. N. (1938). *Modes of Thought.* New York: Free Press, 1966.

Whitehead, A. N. (1948). *Essays in Science and Philosophy.* New York: Philosophical Library.

Winnicott, D. (1958). *Through Paediatrics to Psycho-Analysis.* New York: Basic Books.

Winnicott, D. (1965). *The Maturational Processes and the Facilitating Environment: Studies in the Theory of Emotional Development.* New York: International Universities Press.

Winnicott, D. (1971). *Playing and Reality.* London: Routledge.

Winnicott, D. (1986). *Holding and Interpretation.* New York: Grove.

Winnicott, D. (1989). *Psychoanalytic Explorations.* Cambridge, MA: Harvard University Press.

Wittgenstein, L. (1953). *Philosophical Investigations* (3rd ed., G. Anscombe, Trans.). New York: Macmillan.

Wittgenstein, L. (1921). *Tractatus Logico-Philosophicus* (D. Pears & D. McGuinness, Trans.). Atlantic Highlands, NJ: Humanities Press, 1961.

Wolf, E. (1988). *Treating the Self: Elements of Clinical Self Psychology.* New York: Guilford Press.

Zucker, H. (1993). Reality: Can it be only yours or mine? *Contemporary Psychoanalysis, 29,* 479–486.

Index

Pragmatism, 83
Pragmatist shift to meaning, 146–147
Pragmatist view of misunderstanding, 141–158
Prejudice, 69–71, 72, 73, 108
Prereflective unconsciousness, 79–80
Primary selfobject relatedness, 175–179, 203
Process
  experience as, 54, 177
  relatedness as, 177
Product, 54
Protagoras, 57–58
Prototypic memories, 114–115
Psychoanalysis
  certainty in, 48–51
  critique of positivism within, 46–48
  efficacy of, 160–171
  and philosophy, 2–4
  theory-choice in. *See* Theory-choice
  truth and reality in, 142–147
Psychoanalytic accounts, of Schreber, since Freud, 189–193
Psychoanalytic fallibilism. *See* Fallibilism
Psychoanalytic theory, 142
  experience in, 76–82
Psychoanalytic understanding, 23–24, 171
  healing through, 159–179
  intersubjectivity and self psychology and, 7, 9, 10, 11
  meaning and, 148–151
Psychoanalytic work, on affect, 90–95
Psychosomatic illness, 111–112

R

Radical empiricism, 84
Rationality, theory-choice and, 34–36
Realism, 27, 29
  objectivism versus, 58–62
  perspectival, 2, 3–4, 53–62, 75, 149, 158
  scientific, 76, 77, 78, 81, 84, 144

Reality, in psychoanalysis, 29, 142–147
Reasonable criteria, for theory-choice, 40–43
Reasonableness, philosophy and, 36–40
Relatedness and developmental understanding, 27–29
  of emotional life, 95, 96, 97–99, 102, 103–104
  as process, 177
  selfobject, primary and derivative, 175–179, 203
  understanding as, 15, 23, 24
Relational experience, of Schreber, 193–199
Relativism, 3, 4, 10, 29, 52
  subjectivism versus, 56–58
Renik, O., 71, 131
Repetition, 29, 109
  dread of, 139
Representational remembering, 110
Resistance, 29, 75
Response, 22–23
Ricoeur, P., 16
RIGs (representations of interactions generalized), 80, 114, 115
Rilke, R., 6
Roethke, T., 105
Ruptures. *See* Misunderstanding
Ryle, G., 121

S

Sadness, 201–202
Schafer, R., 26, 62, 77, 78, 144, 146
Schatzman, M., 190–191
Schleiermacher, F., 69, 70, 72–73
Schreber, D. P., 180–205
  efforts of, at self-restoration, 202–205
  Freud's account of, 185–189
  and his memoirs, 182–184
  psychoanalytic accounts of, since Freud, 189–193
  relational experience of, 193–199
  self-experience of, 199–202
Schwaber, E., 71, 181

Lightning Source UK Ltd.
Milton Keynes UK
22 January 2010